D0760695

Diagnosis: Difference

The Moral Authority
of Medicine

Abby L. Wilkerson

Cornell University Press

Ithaca and London

First published 1998 by Cornell University Press
First printing, Cornell Paperbacks, 1998

Printed in the United States of America

Library of Congress Cataloging-in-Publication Data

Wilkerson, Abby L. (Abby Lynn), 1958–
    Diagnosis : the moral authority of medicine / Abby L. Wilkerson.
        p.   cm.
    Includes index.
    ISBN 0-8014-3448-3 (alk. paper). — ISBN 0-8014-8459-6 (pbk. : alk. paper)
        1. Women—Health and hygiene—United States—Sociological aspects.
    2. Women's Health services—Political aspects—United States.   3. Feminism—
    Health aspects—United States.   I. Title.
    RA778.2.W54   1998
    306.4′61′082973—dc21   98-8217
                                                                                    CIP

Cornell University Press strives to use environmentally responsible suppliers and materials to the fullest extent possible in the publishing of its books. Such materials include vegetable-based, low-VOC inks and acid-free papers that are also recycled, totally chlorine-free, or partly composed of nonwood fibers.

Cloth printing   10 9 8 7 6 5 4 3 2 1
Paperback printing   10 9 8 7 6 5 4 3 2 1

Diagnosis: Difference

for

Pat and Lauren

whose love inspires, challenges, and comforts me

and for Cindy, Silvana, Dan, Sammie, Lisa, and Peg

some of the smartest, funniest,

and most amazing people in the world

Contents

Acknowledgments

I began this project at the University of Illinois at Chicago, where I received invaluable help from a number of people. I want to thank Sandra Bartky for her perceptive readings and advice at earlier stages of this work, her strong support and encouragement, and all the Lake Michigan picnics. (Tortellini salad without the sand just isn't the same.) Timothy Murphy took an early interest in my work, and I have benefited greatly from his guidance, meted out with humor and style. Charles Mills also posed a number of insightful questions which proved invaluable to me in the process of research and writing. Peg Strobel, Alice Dan, and Neal Grossman provided useful bibliographical suggestions. I also thank Valerie McQuay and Charlotte Jackson for their support and friendship.

At Texas Tech University, my first philosophy teacher, Danny Nathan, showed me that philosophy could change people's lives. He continues to be an example to me as a teacher, thinker, and friend.

I am greatly indebted to many friends and colleagues in the English department at George Washington University. I thank Chris Sten, chair of the department, for generously providing manuscript assistance funds, and Connie Kibler and Lucinda Kilby for their support. Pam Presser, Jon White, Jill Ehnenn, Cayo Gamber, and Nancy Whichard read and commented on parts of this manuscript; their generous and insightful responses helped me enormously. I have enjoyed a productive and inspiring relationship with other members of the Queer Theory Group and the Writing Program, especially Dan Moshenberg, YouMe Park, Robin Meader, Jamie Peacock, Stacy Wolf, Debbie Bruno, and Bob McRuer.

Alison Shonkwiler, my editor at Cornell University Press, has given me many perceptive and useful responses to this project; working with her has been an inspiration and a pleasure. Carrie Brecke and Durrell Dew helped in important ways at different stages of this process. Samantha Brennan and Joyce Carpenter read and discussed early versions of the manuscript with me (and made exemplary contributions to potlucks when we were graduate students in Chicago). Marilyn Carlander provided a number of useful resources, and kept stubbornly insisting on paying attention to difference long before it was fashionable. Deb DeBruin's rationalism seminar, and her responses to early versions of my work, influenced my thinking in productive ways. I thank Jenny Faust, Bob Blume, Carolyn Kotlarski, and the students in my AIDS seminar at UIC for many interesting conversations; my English 10 and 11 students at George Washington also have provided lively discussions of sexuality, culture, and health. Lisa Heldke read the manuscript attentively; every writer should have a friend, reader, and colleague so insightful and supportive. Thanks to Lauren Kneisly and BARF (Bisexual and Radical Feminists) for inspiration. The women of Maryland NARAL (National Abortion Rights Action League) provided anti-racism training, pizza, rousing political discussions, and my first sense of community in the D.C. area. Silvana Gambardella also read part of the manuscript and made many thoughtful comments about the health care system. Lisa Winter kindly shared her daughter Diana's story.

A portion of Chapter 1 appears in my essay "'Her Body Her Own Worst Enemy': The Medicalization of Violence against Women," in *Violence against Women: Philosophical Perspectives,* ed. Stanley G. French, Wanda Teays, and Laura M. Purdy (Ithaca: Cornell University Press, 1998). Part of Chapter 2 appears in my article "Homophobia and the Moral Authority of Medicine," *Journal of Homosexuality* 27.3/4 (1994): 329–47.

After all these years, I want to thank Glen Hunt. As my high school government (not civics) teacher, he took my rather incoherent political opinions seriously while gently pushing me toward new information. He has given up on corrupting the youth of Idalou, Texas, with his liberal ways, and is now working on infiltrating the Texas legislature.

My partner, Pat McGann, has influenced my thinking in more ways than I can say (and is a terrific reader and editor). My daughter Lauren is almost always ready for a philosophical conversation, and even likes to read my work: a mother's dream. I thank my brother Chris and sister Wendy, the West family, and the McGann family for their support, as well as the Jenkinses. At Ellie's Garden, "Women's Books and More," Linda McGann and Wanda Clark provided a haven, along with many essential readings.

Finally, I want to express my gratitude to my mother, Margaret Wilkerson, and my late father, Bill Wilkerson, who taught me through their example about the importance of having convictions and standing up for them. I only hope the end result is not too alarming.

A. L. W.

Diagnosis: Difference

Introduction: Activism, Health, and Scholarship

In recent years the consumer, women's health, and AIDS movements have vividly demonstrated both the urgency of various groups' health care needs and the shortcomings of medicine with regard to their treatment. In the 1970s and 1980s, feminists, lesbians, gay men, and bisexuals extended their identity politics to activism focusing on health and the politics of health care (see Phelan 1989). While the feminist movement is credited with more extensive theorizing of the politics of health care, the gay liberation movement was also quick to choose medicine as a prime target for change (Altman 1987, 93–94). Members of oppressed and marginalized groups experienced mistreatment and neglect by health care professionals and institutions, often owing to bias against these groups, as well as to ignorance about them and their needs. Medicine also played a critical role in the "naturalization" of an inferior status socially attributed on the basis of gender or sexual orientation. Activists were concerned with exposing the ways in which medicine reinforced other aspects of social disadvantage, or even created new disadvantages of its own, but at the same time with securing access to health care, improving the quality of that care for women and others, transforming the structure of the health care professions, and increasing the participation of disadvantaged groups in the field. Activists also raised important new questions about the relationship of health care to sexual diversity and autonomy.[1] Finally, activists

I

brought attention to the ill health consequences of oppression and targeted health as one of the main arenas for social change.

In this book I use the tools of feminist philosophy, cultural studies, and queer theory to contribute to a new understanding of the relationship between health and justice. My aim is both critical and constructive. I argue that standard philosophical conceptions of this relationship fail to address the needs of oppressed social groups adequately, thus overlooking significant injustices and reinforcing a status quo in which some are privileged at others' expense. On this view, analyses of justice in the realm of health must incorporate concepts of oppression and social group differentials in order to weigh the needs of all; in addition, the standpoints of oppressed groups offer insights that can foster widely beneficial changes in health care.

Two aspects of this project in particular are fairly uncommon in the philosophical literature: I examine the discourses of medicine and bioethics together, in order to indicate the continuities of thought whereby a simplistic dichotomy between the natural and the social occurs in both discourses, with inegalitarian consequences; and I use the perspectives of women of various sexual orientations, together with those of gay and bisexual men, to reveal the significant role of oppressive sexual and reproductive ideologies—whether implicit or explicit—in medicine and bioethics. These continuities are problematic for an additional reason. Not only are the two discourses ostensibly free of ideological influences (or at least they aim to be so), but also they are perceived to be autonomous of each other, each relying on its own distinct conceptual foundations and justificatory schemes—an independence that is required in order for bioethics to fulfill its function, the moral evaluation of medicine and health care. It is clear that the discipline of bioethics cannot evaluate the ideological influences of medicine if it shares them to a significant degree.

Situating applied ethics discussions in the context of activist movements provides a concrete focus in the self-identified, urgent concerns of many people at the present time. I see addressing such concerns as a legitimate and valuable service for philosophy to provide; moreover, I believe that the passionate interest in policy issues of those most directly affected ought to play an important role in policy decisions. In particular I address the women's health and AIDS movements, and the broader identity politics of feminism and of lesbian, gay, and bisexual liberation which gave birth to these groups' health activism. These movements raise important questions about health and justice, including specific critiques of medicine not usually generated within a mainstream liberal framework.

I share certain basic beliefs with other participants in movements against oppression, recognizing, first, that in this society some groups are generally better off than others, and analyzing these differences in welfare as systemic. Factors involved in such assessments may include income, access to education and housing, physical and emotional health, vocational opportunities, mobility, freedom from discrimination, and personal safety, among others. Second, anti-oppression activists typically reject prevailing meritocratic accounts of discrepancies in levels of well-being between social groups, a rejection captured in the phrase "blaming the victim." On this view, the misfortune of one group in relation to another cannot be explained away as the failure of individuals or of the group as a whole; instead, any such general misfortune must have external causes in the social system, including cultural as well as legal and economic forces. And third, anti-oppression activists take the prescriptive stance that the systemic advantage of one group over another is wrong, because it is a key form of injustice that causes profound harms to many people. Thus, we call for the transformation of social relations in order to remedy injustice.

In keeping with this general outlook, one of the starting points of my work is the belief that in contemporary U.S. society (and elsewhere), groups of people are oppressed on the basis of factors such as gender, race, sexual orientation, disability, and economic class.[2] Since this belief is central to this work, it is necessary for me to address some important features of the concepts of oppression and social groups.

I espouse a widely used concept of oppression, articulated persuasively by Marilyn Frye (1983) and Iris Young (1990). On this view, suffering can be attributed to oppression when three crucial elements are present. First, the harms must be multiple, acting together to worsen one's overall situation significantly and limit one's range of options. Second, the practices, beliefs, or acts in question must be pervasive and institutionalized in society—thus distinguishing oppression from disadvantage, which need not be systemic in order to count as such. Third, the harms must accrue differentially to members of a particular social group. From this perspective, an act, belief, or practice need not be intended to oppress in order to do so; what counts is its net effect on members of a particular social group as it functions in people's lives to improve the lot of some while worsening the lot of others. Of course, not everyone agrees with this view. My hope, however, is that this book will contribute to a dual goal: a better understanding of the activist outlook, which most readers would surely agree is an increasingly important influence in the social world, despite conflicting views on the value of that influence; and ultimately conversation and negotiation among people of diverse political viewpoints.

Iris Young defines a social group as "a collective of people who have affinity with one another because of a set of practices or way of life; they differentiate themselves from or are differentiated by at least one other group according to these cultural forms" (1990, 187). Her examples include women, men, American Indians, Latinos, lesbians, and gay men, reflecting the fact that social groups are not distinct and separate from one another, but rather people belong to several groups at once.

I use these concepts of oppression and social groups to draw attention to the meanings and consequences of beliefs and practices as they are connected to the larger social context. It is my belief that medicine and bioethics must be evaluated in their multiple relations to an inegalitarian social context in order to detect and to remedy injustices in the realm of health and medicine. This is an intricate web of relationships, with influences extending to and from each of these elements which connect with and reinforce one another.

I focus on women and gay and bisexual men, attempting to understand them as complex social groups. I attempt to avoid monolithic constructions of "Woman" or "Homosexual," which often function, for instance, to privilege the experiences of the white middle class while excluding people of color and working-class people. Women are oppressed on the basis of gender, yet with different manifestations in different contexts. Anyone who experiences multiple forms of oppression may find it difficult or impossible to determine whether a particular predicament has occurred on the basis of race or of gender, for example. Moreover, not only can multiple forms of oppression coexist in a person's life, but also oppression can coexist with privilege: gay and bisexual men, for example, can be understood to be oppressed on the basis of sexual orientation, despite the gender privilege they may share to the extent that they do not flout conventional norms of masculinity.

Typically, activists in the women's and lesbian, gay, and bisexual movements are committed to opposing oppression on the basis of their own self-described identity.[3] This political grounding in the direct personal experience of oppression can foster a profound understanding of injustice rooted in subjective, personal experience. Taking this outlook as a point of departure, I hope to contribute both to the ongoing critique of objectivity construed as detachment, and to the defense of both situated and subjective modes of knowledge.[4]

Identity and experience, however, are not always infallible guides, given that oppressive beliefs may be internalized by members of oppressed groups, or turned against others. Moreover, as lesbian feminist theorist Elly Bulkin articulates so clearly, identity very often is a matter of privilege as well as oppression: "How much easier it is for someone to say simply that she is oppressed . . . and not to examine the various forms of privilege which so often co-exist with an individual's oppression" (Bulkin, Pratt, and Smith 1984, 99). She and her coauthors, Minnie Bruce Pratt and Barbara Smith, are especially concerned with subtle as well as overt racism and anti-Semitism among feminists. Thus they, along with other activists in the women's and the lesbian, gay, and bisexual movements, call for a critical awareness of the ways in which identity may give one a stake in the perpetuation of one form of oppression, simultaneous with one's opposition to other forms.[5]

During the same period in which these forms of identity politics and health activism emerged, critics were beginning to explore the implications of these socially engaged perspectives for academic discourse. The philosophical discipline of bioethics began to address not only highly specific moral problems in medicine (Buchanan 1981, 3) but the broader relation between justice and health care as well. Laurence B. McCullough notes widespread social inequality with respect to health care, an important theme in the literature: "The present health care system is riddled with inequalities. Unfair advantages are accruing to individuals or groups of individuals on the basis of such factors as race, economic status, geo-

graphical location, and age. . . . [T]he present arrangements for the organization and delivery of and access to health care in our society are unjust
and in need of reform" (1981, 52–53).

Along with a "burgeoning of bioethics" (Buchanan 1981, 3), feminism and postmodernism were emerging as critical academic frameworks
which would undermine the supposed humanism of Western philosophical ideals. They challenged the universalist tradition of the Enlightenment, with its focus on liberty, equality, and individual rights: how strong
was its power to liberate when some groups were still disadvantaged after centuries of "enlightened" Western civilization? The social critiques
generated by these theoretical outlooks suggest that the methodologies
of rationalist liberal philosophy had failed to embody the values of that
tradition.

These important critiques—which apply in varying ways to the dominant framework of mainstream moral philosophy, political philosophy,
and applied ethics, including bioethics—provide valuable tools for analyzing and critiquing social phenomena. The philosopher Susan Sherwin
argues that an explicitly political analysis must be incorporated into bioethics, addressing feminist concerns in particular (1989, 1992). In my view,
bioethics has been most attentive to disadvantage in economic terms; thus
traditional access issues directly related to income are considered far more
often than issues of gender and sexual orientation or cultural influences on
medicine and health. For this reason I second Sherwin's assessment that a
feminist and sexually inclusive analysis has much to offer medical ethics.

A great deal of important and interesting recent work theorizes the
philosophical meanings of social difference in the context of health. Feminists have applied their insights to specific issues, especially reproduction, and have begun to address broader concerns as well.[6] Work from a
gay-affirmative perspective has also begun to appear, addressing AIDS in
particular: philosophers Timothy Murphy (1988, 1991, 1992, 1993) and
Richard Mohr (1988) address the treatment of gay persons with AIDS
within the framework of justice. Annette Dula and Sara Goering offer a
wealth of material on African American health and illness (1994), while
Susan Wendell provides an illuminating account of disability as difference
(1996). This inspiring body of work has prepared the way for broader
philosophical and bioethical reflection on health as an issue of social jus-

tice, assessing the needs of all groups in a more inclusive way and using neglected perspectives as a resource for change. In order for this change to occur, however, underlying conceptual issues in mainstream philosophical methodology must be addressed.

Liberal moral and political theory tends to concern itself with the interactions of persons as rational subjects. Within this framework, what makes these persons free agents, and in some sense rough equals despite their differences, is their possession of the capacity for reason. Bioethics operates within this larger tradition, yet focuses on interactions where that rough equality, and thus the balance of power, is upset: by the frailties of human illness, and by the advantage of doctors over patients owing to their professional and class status as well as to the neediness inherent in patienthood. Susan Sherwin praises medical ethics' concern for the quality of doctor-patient relationships and its recognition of the potential for harm in power imbalances therein (1989). The field's illumination of this risk to autonomy and personhood has been a great achievement, starting from the basic rationalist assumptions of liberalism, which are then considered within a particular context where the interactions of persons as free agents are threatened.

What the discipline of medical ethics does not widely do is question these basic assumptions. Feminist critics have charged that the presumed neutrality of liberal theory actually functions to obscure a pervasive bias, reflecting the gender, class, race, and sexual norms of our society rather than achieving a "view from nowhere" (Nagel 1986); and that liberalism's detached mode of analysis should be replaced with a model of dialogue and negotiation between parties who represent their own interests.[7]

Without careful attention to these issues, bioethics risks the same charges of bias. These critiques raise significant questions of oppression and social group difference which have gone largely unexplored in bioethics, and are important from multiple disciplinary standpoints. Bioethics represents a unique interface between humanities and medical science, fostering much-needed interdisciplinary dialogue in medical schools and in clinical and even policy or legislative settings. For cultural studies scholars, who sometimes lament the difficulty of bringing cultural analysis to public conversations outside the academy,[8] bioethics presents a strategic opportunity to use these tools in the service of material change. At the same time, bioethicists must become aware that social group difference is not marginal but central to our work. When we fail to attend to its manifestations, we run the risk of violating many of the ideals that are central to the profession, despite our best intentions.

A wealth of literature on gender and sexuality,[9] including social science and interdisciplinary work in women's health,[10] as well as work in poststructuralist and psychoanalytic schools of film theory, cultural studies, and feminist theory,[11] illuminates the "material-semiotic" character of the body, health, and illness.[12] Although there are numerous controversies between and within these fields, the shared assumption is that human experience is always mediated through culture. Biology, then, is neither deterministic nor autonomous from culture, but in constant interaction with culture. Moreover, any aspect of human experience and culture—including the expert discourse of medicine, along with popular representations of the body, gender, and sexuality—can be read as a text that expresses the large and small workings of power relationships within a given society. Cultural representations and norms have material effects; physicality, and human biology itself, exist in dynamic relation to social practice. The advantage of this perspective for exploring the relation between health and justice is its illumination of the body as a political site, and of health and disease, sexuality and gender, as culturally mediated phenomena which are always expressions of social values. Such a material-semiotic analysis offers important resources for bioethical reflection on bodily experience, as well as the nonrational influences behind, and the sociopolitical character of, medical discourse itself.

I propose, then, to explore the advantages for bioethics of an approach that (1) identifies health as an issue of justice;[13] (2) advocates the distinct interests of women; (3) advocates the distinct interests of lesbians, gay men, and bisexuals; (4) attends carefully to the complex and multiple nature of these groups; (5) situates its analysis in the politics of those movements; and (6) utilizes interdisciplinary methods of cultural analysis and a material-semiotic conception of health, "produced jointly and reflexively by (universal) biology and (particular) society" (Jordan 1983, 1).

Analytic philosophers tend to construe the relation between health and justice in terms of the allocation of resources and the distribution of access to health care—clearly a pressing issue. Yet in the views of some activists and critics, many aspects of the relation between health and justice cannot readily be addressed within these constraints. I develop this claim by exploring philosophers David Gauthier's (1983) and Norman Daniels's (1985) treatments of the relation between justice and health. Their theories of access to health care differ in ways that are significant for members of disadvantaged groups. Nonetheless, they share a tendency to minimize or misunderstand common issues in the health of women, and other difficulties in considering the interests of oppressed groups.

Feminist and postmodernist critiques of prevailing contractarian theories of justice raise serious concerns about what is omitted from these theories. For example, the Rawlsian framework of justice can be seen to exclude the "private" or "personal," so that gender and family relations are not a concern of justice. Seyla Benhabib argues that John Rawls's "original position" method of promoting objectivity in hypothetical deliberation on social arrangements actually reflects and reinforces white male privilege.[14] Thus she substitutes "the standpoint of the concrete other," replacing hypothetical reflection with actual dialogue as a means of addressing diverse interests (Benhabib 1986). In response, Nancy Fraser contends that dialogue and negotiation must involve representation on the basis of "group identity" rather than "unique individuality" or "universal humanity" (1986, 428).

The philosopher Iris Young argues that a major failure of most liberal theories of justice is their reliance on the "distributive paradigm," which she sees as the operative principle of most treatments of justice in applied ethics as well, including medical ethics (1990, 19). Many important social goods, she argues, cannot readily be understood as a kind of "stuff" which society can allot more or less of to individuals. For example, the cultural representation of a group is not well captured by the distributive paradigm. Young argues that this paradigm of justice functions to obscure significant and widespread harms experienced by some disadvantaged groups in society, such as homophobia (on the level of individual psychology as well as at the level of broader cultural frameworks), which is particularly difficult to address within the constraints of the distributive paradigm of justice. Young recognizes oppression as a key aspect of injustice, widening the scope of analysis beyond the distributive paradigm to include aspects of oppression such as cultural imperialism,[15] exploitation, marginalization, violence, and powerlessness. She advocates "a general principle that promotes attending to group differences in order to undermine oppression" (12). I find this framework far more able than the distributive paradigm to capture the ways in which injustice is interwoven into the social structure (as I argue throughout this book), rather than simply happening to befall some unfortunate individuals.

This charge to look beyond issues of allocation and distribution can be applied fruitfully to an examination of medical constructions of women's bodies and specific health issues, as well as medical constructions of the relationship between sexuality and HIV transmission, and more broadly to the role of medicine in the perpetuation and legitimation of sexism and homophobia.

On the face of it, medical discourse and mainstream conceptualizations of social justice serve quite different purposes, yet both are used in the attempt to produce just and beneficial public policy. The discourse of social justice (which I take to encompass a broad political spectrum, and to include popular discourse as well as social and political philosophy) is used in the moral evaluation of public policy, as when we ask: Is this course of action compatible with the requirements of justice? Medical discourse in the form of concepts, values, and "facts" shapes questions such as: Is this course of action medically sound? How will it affect public health?

Despite the attempt to employ each discourse in the service of just and beneficial public policy, however, their influence has not always been egalitarian. The realm of medicine is presumed to be value-free; yet not only has it been used as an instrument of oppression against lesbians, gays, and bisexuals,[16] but also it has served as an ideological support for other forms of oppression—for example, judging and punishing women for sexual behavior deemed immoral (Sherwin 1992, 213–16).

Inegalitarian influences can also be found in the discourse of justice. Iris Young argues that the prevailing distributive formulation (despite great concern for objectivity) obscures significant harms which systematically accrue to members of disadvantaged groups such as gay people. Obscuring such harms may even reinforce social callousness toward the suffering of these groups and a lack of will to remedy these harms in the name of justice. Significantly, the discourses of medicine and justice share the central epistemic principle of objectivity construed as detachment—a value hotly contested in recent and influential work in feminist theory, epistemology, and philosophy of science.[17] I find that lesbian and gay experiences with medicine also raise questions about the value of this principle, at least as it is typically construed and employed, and that these questions are an important concern for bioethics.

In the first two chapters I evaluate the discourse of medicine in two contexts. In Chapter 1 I explore the medicalization of women's health, focusing particularly on violence against women, menstruation, and childbirth, areas where medicine stigmatizes women and expresses conservative norms about relationships with others, resulting in an erasure of women's sense of self. I also defend the appropriateness and necessity of *just* moral commitments in medicine, as exemplified by feminist work in health care. In Chapter 2 I continue to explore medical stigmatizing and moralizing in the context of AIDS, and offer a characterization of four significant aspects of medicine, most of which have not been adequately addressed in bioethics.

I then turn to bioethics discourse, where access to health care exemplifies the necessity of addressing all aspects of medicine, although typically some are neglected. In Chapter 3 I explore the nature of health care as a social good, while in Chapter 4 I examine the descriptive account of health and its role in theories of access to health care.

It must be acknowledged that I bring to this exploration my own subjectivity, my own social location—as a participant in the movements I describe, as a teacher and mother, and as a bisexual feminist. Simultaneously I am drawn to holistic notions of health, cautious of medical intervention, and yet aware of my own reliance on the institution of medicine. More than once as the following pages have accumulated, I have been absorbed in Foucault's illumination of "the clinic" as the site of power relations, indeed, of ever-increasing surveillance and control of daily life (1975), while at the same time I found myself facing the very problems I was attempting to theorize.

As I worked on this project, my brother Chris Wilkerson learned that he had colon cancer, the disease that proved fatal to our father. Later, a fall from a horse crushed three sections of Chris's vertebrae and fractured a fourth. During this time I also learned of my own precancerous polyps, and of the technology for treating this condition, which is surely one of the success stories of modern medicine. These were just some of the health crises arising during this project which never let me forget both the value of access to health care and the experiential side of policy issues — the long nights when one of Chris's surgeries resulted in complications, our fears and anxieties. This confessional moment is not simply a statement of the unavoidable influence of subjectivity and personal circumstance. Instead, it expresses my awareness that I, like others, am situated in the conflict at the heart of this work: the urgent demand for a good that is in many ways problematic, yet one that I am grateful is available to me and to those I love.

I

Her Body Her Own Worst Enemy: The Medicalization of Women's Health

At some point in our lives, most women in contemporary U.S. society seek health care for reasons related to menstruation, menopause, pregnancy, childbirth, or violence. The last element may seem out of place, especially if one thinks of it as socially influenced in a way that the others, which may be perceived as more "biological" in nature, are not. I do not mean to suggest by including it here that violence against women is biologically ordained or inevitable in any way. I advocate a material-semiotic approach to women's health which resists the dichotomy between biology and culture, recognizing that biology is inseparable from social practices, representations, meanings. In this respect, those health care needs that might be considered to arise biologically in the female life cycle are similar to sexual assault or domestic violence: their manifestations in women's bodies, minds, and lives are thoroughly embedded within particular social contexts.

Not only do most women have some contact with the health care system around at least one of these issues, but also they serve as excellent examples of the medicalization of women's life experiences. Twenty percent of women recently surveyed report having been raped, while 12 percent of girls report having been sexually abused, and 17 percent report physical abuse.[1] Generally, even women who have neither given birth nor experienced rape or battery must nonetheless reconcile themselves in some

13

way to these issues as important features of the social world, influencing women's views of ourselves and how we are viewed and treated by others. For this reason alone, it is important to understand the impact of the medicalization of these experiences.

A further reason is found in the embeddedness of health care in its social context, despite its attempts to transcend this supposedly serious limitation. Neither practitioners, institutions, nor medical knowledge can be immune to social influence. Medical theory and practice stigmatize these bodily experiences common to women, and thus femaleness itself, as if women were defective males.[2] Medicine legitimizes a characterization of female selflessness as both an implicit behavioral norm and an existential categorization, an ideology that can deeply affect a woman's sense of herself and her efficacy in the world.

Medicine also conceptualizes the woman patient as white, heterosexual, middle class, able-bodied, young, and HIV negative. The many women who depart from this norm may find themselves patronized, controlled, neglected, punished, dehumanized, and even criminalized by the institution of medicine. If medicine implicitly understands femaleness as selflessness and conceptualizes women patients in terms of social privilege, then women of color, lesbians and bisexual women, women with disabilities, working-class and poor women, older women, and HIV-positive women are likely to be marginalized at best, or treated as constitutionally incapable of the selflessness that is womanhood, and therefore in need of control by others.

This norm of selflessness operates in many ways: erasing women's subjectivities; alienating women from our own bodies; erasing and undermining women's agency; erasing women's interests as they are distinct from others'; and eroding women's self-regard as well as our identification with and regard for other women. Paradoxically, medicine simultaneously relegates women to the category of Other as it radically individualizes us. Oppressive social relations are presented as facts of nature, taking biological essence as the basis for implicit relational norms which define women in relation to others rather than as beings in our own right. At the same time, being treated as pathologically outside this norm leaves one vulnerable to neglect or to harsh sanctions, although it may also make one more suspicious of medical control and thus more capable of resisting it, as Dorothy Roberts has argued is the case for women of color (1994).

My critique of medicine's inegalitarian treatment of women is based on these central tenets of the women's health movement:

1. A social context of patriarchy, racism, classism, and homophobia is harmful to women's health.

2. The health care system as presently structured reflects and reinforces society's devaluation of women.[3]

3. To address these two problems adequately, not only must they be understood within this social context, but the social structure must be transformed in many ways as well.

4. Thus, health care must incorporate the goal of promoting women's interests and agency, as workers, professionals, and clients, in medical (and other) contexts.

I find that this perspective offers two distinct yet related advantages over more traditional medicine: it contributes to "better science," more accurate descriptions or understandings of physiological states and processes and the contexts in which they occur, and thus a better basis for medical treatment; and it facilitates medicine that is morally preferable in its conceptualization and treatment of women and its potential to rectify some aspects of an oppressive social context. Thus, my opposition to certain normative commitments in medicine, rather than being a critique of all such medical norms, is part of a broader defense of *just* norms. Recognizing that medicine is a material-semiotic phenomenon because it too is embedded in its social context leads to the possibility that it can be responsive to that context.

I begin with an overview of the mainstream medical paradigm, focusing on the ways in which it obscures or excludes some important considerations, with inegalitarian consequences.[4] I then examine the influence of this paradigm on current theory and practice in women's health.

The Mainstream Medical Paradigm

Over the past few decades, a diverse group of consumer activists and radical academics, including ACT UP (Crimp 1988), the Boston Women's Health Book Collective (1992), Mary Daly (1978), Angela Davis (1981), Barbara and John Ehrenreich (1970), Gay Men's Health Crisis of New York (Kayal 1993), Ivan Illich (1977), and Thomas Szasz (1974), have critiqued the U. S. health care system. Many of these critics are particularly concerned with the role of medicine in justifying, reinforcing, or contributing directly to specific forms of oppression—heterosexism, sexism, classism, racism, ageism, and so on—which are elsewhere and otherwise pervasive in society.

One form of this sociopolitical role of medicine has been called "medicalization," which the social critic Ivan Illich describes as a "medical and paramedical monopoly over hygienic methodology and technology . . . a device to convince those who are sick and tired of society that it is they who are ill, impotent, and in need of technical repair" (1977, xvii). "Medicalization," in short, is a way of understanding a broad array of human behaviors and problems as the pathologies of specific organisms. I illustrate this concept in a historical context, where it is most easily understood, to set the stage for more current manifestations.

Certain diagnoses historically applied to women are prime examples of medicalization. The historian Karl Figlio argues, contrary to popular opinion, that the development of medical theory in the nineteenth century was structured as much by political need as by progress in verifying scientific hypotheses and applying them to alleviate suffering (1983). Figlio demonstrates how moral and political norms were codified in the nineteenth-century concept of chlorosis. Medical scientists based this diagnosis on certain chemical blood changes such as anemia, and linked it to the supposed idleness of female adolescence, despite the fact that many "chlorotics" were working class and wage earners at an early age. Called "the virgin's disease," chlorosis was "associated . . . with disappointed sexual feelings," and the standard treatment regimen—"early hours, regularity, open air, exercise, controlled diet and emotional life—was wholesomely childlike" (221).

This diagnostic category constructed female physiology through the social norm of feminine delicacy and sexual purity. Construing adolescence as a stage of idleness, especially for girls, obscured the social practices that created leisure for daughters of privileged men while treating working-class girls as cheap labor sources, thereby "deflecting criticism from socioeconomic conditions" (229). Figlio also underscores the medical privatization of illness. Disease typologies become patient typologies, "transfer[ring] the locus of pathology from society to the individual" (232).

The sociopolitical function of medicine was also operative in nineteenth-century notions of puerperal or childbed fever. Much less common when female midwives attended women in labor, the fever was actually an assortment of infections, usually caused by the unsanitary practices of male practitioners who had attended other patients with communicable diseases. These male practitioners construed the fever as the sign of a woman's immorality as well as the weakness of the female body. According to the historian Jo Murphy-Lawless, male "midwives" popularized the idea that the fever was "most prevalent among women carrying illegitimate babies . . . [and] that the disturbed psychological state of these women encouraged the fever to take root. . . . Women were forced to bear the responsibility both for their marginalized social status and for their deaths in childbirth" (1988, 186). At the same time, female midwives were characterized as superstitious, dirty, and unskilled. Male practitioners used the fever to justify their involvement in and eventual control over childbirth, pathologizing pregnancy and discrediting female midwives at the same time.[5] Thus, medicalization is also a process of institutionalizing professional interests.

It is tempting to dismiss these examples as quaint reminders of the unfortunate prejudices that medical progress has overcome. Yet medical practice, particularly the interactions of female patients and male physicians, continues to be criticized for promoting moral norms in the guise of medical advice. Medical sociologist Kathy Davis's analysis of four hundred tape recordings of clinical interactions identifies frequent paternalism, with "general practitioners making moral judgments about women's roles as wives and mothers, psychologizing women's problems, not taking their complaints seriously, massive prescription of tranquilizers, [and] usurpation of women's control over their reproduction" (1988, 22). Davis finds this paternalism particularly insidious, given the apparent benevolence of doctors: "It was precisely the intimate, pleasant quality of the medical encounter itself that made issues of power and control seem like something else" (22).

In my view, the function of medicine as power and control depends not only on the social roles of doctor and patient but also on the social construction of science as the foundation of modern medicine. This scientific grounding of medicine provides a base of knowledge; but a deeper analysis suggests that the detached, objectivist epistemology of medicine, rather than liberating it from the tyranny of values, instead legitimizes medicine's implicit moral-political judgments.

Michel Foucault's study *The Birth of the Clinic* (1975) clarifies the relationship between the epistemology of medicine and its moral authority, tracing the medicalization of society which transferred the moral domain from the soul onto the body. As the church began to lose its position as sole moral arbiter, a new version of public moral order was needed, and medicine fit the bill. In the modern era of medicine, which Foucault calls "the clinic," its knowledge base shifted from empirical information apprehended directly through the senses to a new mode of quantifiable and precise data made possible by an ever-increasing array of instruments. This was a knowledge that was utterly detached, as far removed as possible from the distortion not only of emotion but of the senses as well. Foucault succinctly states the epistemic principle of the clinic: "That which is not on the scale of the gaze falls outside the domain of possible knowledge" (166). Instead of ordinary human vision, this gaze suggests a mode of knowledge that seemed indisputable owing to its technological grounding (for instruments cannot lie), its precision and quantification, its detachment and objectivity. Thus, by association, the moral and political judgments reflected in medicine gained the status of objective truth as well.

"The scale of the gaze" continues to manifest itself in Donald Seldin's defense of the Flexnerian model of medicine and medical education (1984). In his 1910 report on the state of the profession, Abraham Flexner understood medicine as based strictly in physics, chemistry, biology, and related subdisciplines. Following in Flexner's footsteps, Seldin—a prominent medical administrator, professor, and consultant—limits the role of medicine to the following task: to "bring to bear an increasingly powerful conceptual and technical framework for the mitigation of that type of human suffering rooted in biomedical derangements" (62). According to Seldin, medicine "must by definition become dissociated from concerns of a social nature, the solutions of which lie outside those boundaries" (57). This new instance of detached epistemology combines a sense of the limits of medicine with perhaps a stronger faith in the powers of precise technical knowledge.

This model structures medical discourse at the level of practice as well.

Suzanne Poirier and Daniel Brauner (1988) argue that the objectivity and detachment in "the daily language of medical discourse" obscure the humanistic concerns of patients and doctors: individual values, personalities, relationships, needs, and circumstances. These "nonmedical" aspects of life have great bearing on the subjective experience of illness and healing, and on medical diagnosis and treatment as well.[6] This ejection of humanistic concerns from the daily language of medical discourse reflects the narrow Flexnerian framework. To adapt Foucault's metaphor here, the fact that such concerns are "not on the scale of the gaze" only exacerbates the power imbalances in the interaction of doctor and patient, because the patient's perceptions and desires and other "nonmedical" aspects of health and illness are not necessarily translatable into that discourse.

Violence against Women

The medical treatment of violence against women indicates the harmful consequences of the overly narrow medical paradigm defended by Seldin. Mainstream medicine often treats the symptoms of violence while ignoring and even obscuring the causes, isolating a specific injury from the context in which it occurred and, in the case of domestic violence, is likely to recur; it fails to reduce the risk of medical treatment's retraumatizing patients; and in many cases it also reinscribes conservative notions of women's place. Thus, the paradigm Seldin defends not only is inadequate for the needs of women but also is not altogether as objective, nor as free of moral norms, as it purports to be.

First of all, the clinical paradigm may conceal the nature of the injury. A 1990 *Journal of the American Medical Association* report notes that "only 5 percent of 107 victims of domestic violence at a metropolitan emergency department were identified in the physicians' records as abused" (Parsons 1990). Similarly, Evan Stark and colleagues (1983) show that the nature of domestic violence injuries is likely to be obscured in medical care. Their study identifies features of domestic violence which clearly distinguish it from most other injuries seen in emergency rooms, yet finds that these incidents are far more likely to be considered accidents (187–88).

Unfortunately, another distinguishing feature of domestic violence is that its victims may not be in a position to explain the cause of their injuries. Debbie Burghaus, a social worker in a Chicago area hospital, told a reporter, "A lot of times, the victim isn't going to offer to tell you she was beaten up, because he's [the abuser is] waiting for her in the hall, or she's just not empowered to leave him yet" (Parsons 1990).

Although women are sometimes unable to discuss battering because of fears of retribution from the batterer, at other times they may be prevented by the doctor or other medical professional who is privileged to control communication with patients, a feature of medical interactions which systematically disadvantages battered women when they attempt to speak out.[7] In fact, "providers have found that, contrary to their expectations, women have proven quite willing to admit abuse when asked directly in a nonjudgmental way" (Heise 1994, 245). Such simple measures as including the question "Is the patient a victim of domestic violence?" on all patient charts have been shown to increase identification of cases (Colburn 1996), which is vital for legal corroboration, treatment, support services, and prevention of future incidents.

Understanding circumstances such as the difficulty of leaving an abuser requires knowledge of patients' social and economic circumstances. For example, providers need to recognize that the effects of battering are compounded for those who face other forms of oppression as well, including women of color (Richie and Kanuha 1993) and disabled women (Warshaw 1994). Lack of information is not the only problem here; providers' assumptions may prevent them from understanding the situation. Lesbian abuse survivors treated for injuries have sometimes encountered outright denial that one woman can batter another (Poore 1996). In 1990 Nancy Kathleen Sugg surveyed primary care physicians whose patients were mostly white and middle class, asking "why they didn't intervene in cases of domestic violence" (Nechas and Foley 1994, 146). Some responded that "they so closely identified with them they didn't suspect abuse, which they expected to see among poorer, less educated women" (147). Such assumptions harm all women: if some are expected to be victims, then their abuse may be accepted all too easily, while others are considered immune, and therefore are neglected as well.

Dr. Carole Warshaw of Chicago's Cook County Hospital, an expert in domestic violence, told an interviewer that physicians "see their job as fixing the physical problem, and they don't see the person or their life context as part of the problem, so that's not their job" (Parsons 1990). Warshaw and other feminist analysts call for a broader clinical focus, recognizing the social nature of the problem in order to facilitate prevention and intervention efforts. Given the previous examples, this broadening should include a deconstruction of the myths that may influence providers' understanding of women's needs as patients.

The medical paradigm also hinders prevention and treatment by pathologizing victims and thereby relinquishing medical responsibility. Stark and his associates found that many survivors seeking treatment for injuries received "pseudopsychiatric labels in the medical records such as 'patient with multiple vague medical complaints' or 'multiple symptomatology with psychosomatic overlay'" (1983, 195). Yet battered women have long been known to experience the physical manifestations of chronic stress, such as "severe tension headaches, stomach ailments, high blood pressure, allergic skin reactions, and heart palpitations," along with anxiety and depression (Walker 1979, 61). A woman's body registers the daily battering of her subjectivity, prompting her to seek a medical remedy which may be her only safe outlet for addressing the multiple harms the batterer has inflicted on her. Yet when she attempts to articulate her situation in "the daily language of medical discourse" (Poirier and Brauner 1988, 5), her perceptions are stripped of their meaning. This aspect of medical practice undermines the self-esteem and social authority of women who have been battered. Moreover, psychiatric pathologization not only diverts attention from chronic stress-related illnesses but also fails to address the cause of the problem at all.

This pathologization additionally serves to obscure the group identity of women who are battered, perpetuating the perception that their suffering occurs on a random, individual basis, that it is a case of bad luck rather than a manifestation of relationships between men and women as they are constructed in this society. Participating in support groups with other battered women has helped many to change their lives, learning that they are not alone and that they can begin to exercise greater control over their lives, as other women have done. Fortunately, some hospitals do refer patients identified as battered women to such groups. Every hospital should at the very least refer women to these and other services. Psychiatric pathologization, however, clearly substitutes a diagnosis for real assistance—a diagnosis that can only stigmatize, compounding the hopelessnes and shame that battering often causes (Walker 1979), by eroding women's regard for themselves and other survivors of domestic violence.

Pathologization also serves to mask institutional responsibilities. According to Stark and his colleagues, a survivor who frequently returns to the emergency room may be labeled a chronic complainer or treatment seeker, terms that function "to suppress the 'inappropriate' demands for help of those victimized elsewhere. . . . The label explains the failure of the medical paradigm and the continued suffering of the abused woman in a way that is intelligible, even acceptable, to the physician" (Stark, Flitcraft, and Frazier 1983, 187). They argue convincingly that the medical profession indirectly supports systemic violence against women by failing to acknowledge assault as such, pathologizing the women themselves, who after all enter the hospital seeking health and safety (187). At the same time, this treatment helps to protect the interests of the medical profession in the face of the difficulties the women present.

The failure to identify the cause of an injury may not count as misdiagnosis in the usual sense; yet if domestic violence is perceived as a pattern in a woman's life rather than a series of discrete incidents, a kind of misdiagnosis—and ultimately mistreatment, or inadequate treatment—does occur insofar as symptoms are addressed, but not their underlying causes and their relation to a woman's overall life circumstances. I am not suggesting that providers must single-handedly "cure" these complex social problems, but rather that successful medical treatment requires a close understanding of them. Without this, there are too many stereotypes and false assumptions that can influence providers' interactions with patients at a time when they are traumatized and overwhelmed, and therefore emotionally vulnerable.

One such life circumstance that must be addressed is the economic. Domestic violence is a major cause of poverty for women, which in turn complicates every aspect of domestic violence (Bennett-Haighney 1997, Boodman 1997, Rich 1996). Kristy Woods contends, "A large percentage of homeless women have left home because of domestic violence and frequently must seek medical care for associated injuries" (1994, 106–7). The poor living conditions of homeless women are associated with chronic illness as well—circumstances that must be taken into account if adequate treatment is to be provided. Christine Cassel argues that this situation illustrates the inseparability of "bedside clinical decision making and issues of social justice and resource allocation" (1994, 120). Providers need to realize how economic circumstances may deter women from leaving an abuser, or how poverty and stress may affect the health of women who do. Educated providers will be in a much better position to make connections with available resources and provide appropriate referrals. The medical profession occupies a unique position for advocating the interests of domestic violence survivors, and failing to address economic issues assumes class and gender norms that neglect many women's needs.

A study conducted by Jody Raphael indicates that women who have survived domestic violence or continue to experience it make up the majority of women receiving public assistance. Raphael "documented how domestic violence makes and keeps women poor. Surveys from grassroots welfare-to-work programs around the country revealed the ways in which domestic violence complicates and prolongs the transition from welfare to employment and self-sufficiency" through perpetrators' sabotage and other means (Bennett-Haigney 1997, 5). Caregivers need to be aware of these factors which affect women's health and overall life prospects in order to treat them with the dignity that everyone deserves but is critically important in cases where dignity and self-respect have been jeopardized through violence. Aspects of treatment such as learned sensitivity, referrals, and follow-ups emerge not from detached, "objective" medicine but from socially committed medicine.

The failure to identify and address the total picture, as opposed to the discrete injuries, is also connected to the medical/cultural assumption that heterosexuality and marriage are biologically certified as "natural," hence appropriate, hence safe. This point can be understood by exploring the medical understanding of domestic violence which *is* acknowledged as such. Domestic violence education for the medical profession tends to rely on research on "the violent family," obscuring a widespread social problem by focusing on "an aberrant subtype" of the family rather than "the American family as such" (Stark, Flitcraft, and Frazier 1983, 194). The notion of "the violent family" contains an unstated assumption that "the family" unmodified, with heterosexuality and marriage at its core, is non-violent, a benign institution, where women's physical and financial safety are protected. This language also presents violence as an amorphous cloud hanging over some families, erasing men's agency and control in acts of violence, and pathologizing women and children at the same time.

Here, then, is one manifestation of the relational norms I have alluded to in the medicalization of women's health: the belief that women *belong* in relationships with men, belong in "the family." This normative assumption denies the risks of heterosexuality and family life for women, on a continuum with various forms of violence that affect all women's lives. Furthermore, when violence must be acknowledged, pathologization subtly suggests that somehow the woman must have had a part in it, as a member of a "violent family."

The medicalization of rape also poses difficulties for women. For example, Peter Cartwright's "Sexual Violence" chapter in *Novak's Textbook of Gynecology* (Jones, Wentz, and Burnett 1988) is a well-intentioned yet problematic discussion of the topic.[8] Its influence on medical students is likely to be mixed. On the positive side, Cartwright addresses the relationship of sexual assault to the social context, citing well-known feminist social science literature (528). He also alerts the physician to psychosocial issues that victims face, recommends that physicians take the opportunity to "initiate crisis intervention" (531), and emphasizes the need for "reestablishing the victim's sense of control over her own life situation" (532)—one implication being that victims must be allowed to make their own decisions about whether to report the crime. His obvious concern for women who have been raped is not to be taken for granted in the medical community, given that "many physicians [responding to a survey of personnel in thirty-one Florida emergency rooms] said they felt conducting a forensic rape exam was a waste of their time and expertise" (Nechas and Foley 1994, 146).

Nevertheless, neither Cartwright's treatment of psychosocial issues nor his effort to link rape to the social context is ultimately successful. The physician's first task is the initial interview, which Cartwright alludes to many times, yet specifies neither which questions to ask nor which techniques to use for helping to reduce the survivor's stress during the interview. Cartwright defines medical management of rape to include "the treatment of physical injuries, the prevention of venereal disease and pregnancy, the initiation of crisis intervention, and the collection of forensic specimens and data" (531). For those who have just been violated and traumatized, undergoing this extensive set of procedures is likely to be quite difficult, yet nowhere does Cartwright acknowledge the potential impact of the procedures nor suggest strategies to make them more tolerable.

Furthermore, when Cartwright does address psychosocial issues, he offers very little guidance. The physician is told to ask the woman where she will go after leaving, as well as "how will husband or family view her now that she has been 'violated'" (531), yet he fails to note what sort of answers to look for or how the physician is to respond. Cartwright also recommends a six-week follow-up, at which time the physician is to assess how well the woman is coping and "refer those in need of more intensive therapy" (533). The basis for this assessment, however, is not specified.

Cartwright's discussion of the social context is obviously well intended, its tone sympathetic both to women and to feminist analysis. Yet at a deeper level his writing erases patriarchal agency, individualizes the act of rape as an aberration even as he acknowledges its prevalence, and ultimately pathologizes women themselves. In a section on the "etiology" of rape—a telling example of the medicalization of social relations—Cartwright rejects in one paragraph the claim that the tendency to rape is inherent in males, then provides a one-paragraph discussion of rape "as a social issue," noting that "potential rapists seem quite common in our society" (528). He then proceeds with a five-paragraph examination of individual characteristics of rapists, immediately undercutting the feminist social analysis of rape which he has just cited with seeming approval.

Perhaps the most unsettling passage is the chapter's opening:

> Women are the preferred victims of violence in all societies. Most sexual violence is violence with sexual connotations that is directed toward women. Rape and sexual abuse of women and children is an ancient problem that has plagued all socioeconomic and educational levels in the Western world. Sexual assault is so common in the United States that all women are touched by fear, thinking perhaps they may become a victim. This fear dictates how a woman holds her arms, dresses, or speaks, where she goes and with whom. She knows a misinterpreted gesture may provoke a violent, hateful, perhaps fatal attack upon herself. *Her*

body and her own sexual desires become her own worst enemy. (525; emphasis added)

Note the passive constructions: women are the "preferred victims" of a violence that "is directed toward women" like an approaching thunderstorm, "an ancient problem" that has always "plagued" society, and perhaps will eternally. Cartwright speaks of rape as if it were beyond all human agency or intervention, rather than a conscious, deliberate act by specific men.

In fact, rather than attributing rape to patriarchal male agency, Cartwright presents it as a force emanating from the bodies of women themselves, somehow the consequence of their sexual desires. Surely most rape survivors would be surprised to learn that their own bodies are worse enemies than their assailants. Yet from the perspective of the medical model, the usual suspect is the female body itself, and thus, troubling as this statement may be, it is unsurprising.

Cartwright presents women as tragically and inevitably preoccupied with their own dangerous bodies, as he erases his own gender and physicality, along with that of the doctor or medical student reading his text: the medical view from nowhere. Yet it is exactly this awareness that is vital: not a woman's alleged fear of her own body, but a physician's recognition of the impact of the medical gaze and the medical touch—quite likely a male touch—for a rape survivor. Cartwright's approach to sexual violence exemplifies the confinement of the medical paradigm, which does not extend beyond the boundaries of the patient's body.

The body and desires of the doctor, however, do not cease to exist when they are not acknowledged. Kathryn Morgan writes of physicians who rape their patients, a problem she sees as intractable (1997). Contributing factors include the collusion of other doctors who protect colleagues at the expense of patients, the sense of entitlement that comes with status in a male-dominated profession, a perception of women's bodies as passive objects to be manipulated by physicians, and a complete absence of the kind of self-reflection I have called for.

Another example of the need for medical self-criticism can be found in the situation of women with disabilities. Carol Gill, a disability activist and scholar, says of women and girls with disabilities, "Our social devaluation

places us at high risk for abuse" (1996, 9). Many authors confirm the high
risk of violence for women with disabilities; social isolation and a perceived
lack of credibility exacerbate this vulnerability. "Minority, elderly, lower
socioeconomic, and rural populations" are more likely to experience disabilities, and their lack of status also contributes to the problem (Bernal
1996, 59). Gill asserts the need for health care providers to be especially
alert to signs of violence in women with disabilities (9), yet those who report violence have encountered neglect and denial in health care settings.
Margaret Nosek argues that disabled women's extensive socialization as patients, along with their desexualization by providers and others, increases
their vulnerability dramatically: "There is often dissociation of the self from
the parts of the body being assaulted, rooted in frequent pain inflicted by
doctors and 'helpers,' where privacy is denied, nakedness is the norm, and
women are treated as if they are not human" (1996a, 159). Although women with disabilities are likely to experience this dehumanization to a profound degree that is not always the case for others, they also represent the
conditions of patienthood itself, especially for women. Their experiences
may be unique in certain ways, yet also indicate general failings in the medicalization of violence.

Gynecology

Menstruation and "premenstrual syndrome" are topics of great controversy
in the popular press as well as in the fields of medicine and psychology.[9]
Some researchers note prevalence rates as high as 95 to 97 percent of men-
struating women (Zita 1988, 83–84). Discomfort related to the menstrual
cycle is statistically normal, in the sense that many women experience some
form of it. It is a great leap from this phenomenon, however, to medical
and lay perceptions of cyclical changes as a medical crisis and a sign of female inadequacy. Both perceptions are strongly influenced by the values
and expectations "of a culture that regards the female body as a deficient
version of the real one" (Tavris 1992, 167). Although such overt associations
are surprisingly common, more frequently they are suggested implicitly.
These normative assumptions underlying influential medical notions of the
menstrual cycle seem to require no moral justification, given their pre-

sumed status as medical "facts." A material-semiotic understanding of the menstrual cycle challenges this framework, with distinct advantages for women.

A well-known gynecology text discusses menstruation and menopause as normal, healthy physiological functions, yet describes them in language that conveys pathology and decay. The two main phases of the endometrium (the lining of the uterus) are identified as the "proliferative" and "secretory" phases (Jones, Wentz, and Burnett, 1988, 68). While the two terms may not seem to be overtly evaluative, the authors associate the "proliferation" phase with growth and regeneration, and "secretion" with "rapid loss," "degeneration," and "destruction" (73–76). Similarly, menopause is described in subtly evaluative language: "The menopause (cessation of menses) is undoubtedly due to *failing* ovarian function due to the *exhaustion* of the pool of primary follicles, and the associated decreased steroidogenesis. This, in turn, *disturbs* the pituitary-hypothalamic feedback mechanisms" (398; emphasis added).[10] Such language reflects a sense of older *women* as failing, exhausted, disturbed—as in the familiar situation of accomplished film actresses of forty being rejected for leading roles, while much older men are still considered attractive and distinguished.

This language also reflects the patriarchal definition of women as mothers, existing for the sake of others: when not conceiving, gestating, giving birth, or perhaps lactating, a woman's body is in chaos or even decay, by virtue of the woman's perceived failure to fulfill her body's inherently reproductive design. Femaleness itself becomes a disruptive and dangerous force which must be redeemed by motherhood, or medically subdued and regulated. Older women, apparently, are no longer restrained by the self-lessness of motherhood, and thus in constant danger of degeneracy.

In industrialized capitalist society, health is sometimes conceived of as, or in relation to, production. On this measure, it is women who are likely to be found wanting. The anthropologist Emily Martin identifies the standard "teleological interpretation" of female biology, which defines "menstruation as failed production" (1987, 45) and menopause as the loss of productive capacity. The definition of menopause as "estrogen-deficiency disease" has now become standard.[11] This understanding of female biology, Martin notes, creates a hierarchy in which organic states directly involved in reproduction are "normal" while others are not (41). Menstrual flow is perceived only as the negative indicator that conception did not occur, rather than as a functional process in its own right. That it is (nonpregnant) femaleness itself which is the basis for pathology is evident in the fact that similar states in other parts of the body are not conceptualized analogously. Like menstruation, other organic processes involve the production and secretion of tissue, yet are not perceived as biological "failures": "the lining of the stomach, for example, is shed and replaced regularly, and seminal fluid picks up shedded cellular material as it goes through the various male ducts," yet neither of these processes is understood as "failed production" or waste (Martin 1987, 50).

The economy's influence on gynecological concepts is more than metaphorical. Menstrual cycle research clearly bears the mark of economic and political trends. Carol Tavris's research review demonstrates that the view of menstruation as a problematic and disruptive force in women's lives "comes and goes in phase with women's participation in the labor market" (1992, 139). In the 1930s medical research found that menstrual symptoms posed serious obstacles to women's employment, whereas early in the World War II era, when women's participation in the work force was vital to military and commercial interests, researchers found no such problems. In the 1950s researchers once again found menstruation to interfere with women's functioning in the work force, and in the 1970s, when the number of women in paid employment increased, research on menstruation as disruptive to employment also increased dramatically (Tavris 1992, 139–41).

Premenstrual syndrome, or PMS, is perhaps a unique economic situation in itself. Although some practitioners undoubtedly have the best of motives for treating PMS, it has spawned a major industry which providers and pharmaceutical companies have a large stake in protecting (Tavris 1992, 137–39, 143). Similar claims could be made of many different illnesses, yet PMS offers a distinctive combination of factors: many doctors and laypersons perceive high rates of prevalence, a wide array of markers, and persistence for many years (ensuring many return visits and many prescriptions refilled). It also reflects and reinforces gender stereotypes, which in turn may influence women to perceive their cyclical changes more negatively, and thus to seek treatment; and though no regimen offers a straightforward cure, there are assorted treatments to choose from, which tend not to involve particularly taxing or challenging procedures for the physician. In short, PMS presents a very attractive business opportunity, with strong potential for a serious conflict of interest.

Menstrual pathologization exemplifies the medical norm of female self-lessness, erasing women's distinct interests (moral, political, economic, and otherwise) and subjectivities, even in the understanding of health. From a woman's perspective, neither menstruation nor menopause—as opposed to certain *symptoms* that some women experience—is problematic or unhealthy (or somehow less healthy than pregnancy) in and of itself. Many women who are heterosexually active welcome menstruation as confirming successful contraception and menopause as the end of contraceptive worries (Martin 1987). Gynecology imports the social definition of women as mothers into its concept of female biology. Evaluating women's physiological states in these terms obscures the meaning of menstrual or menopausal health for women apart from the pursuit of childbearing. It also suggests that motherhood is biologically ordained, a natural female state, rather than always culturally mediated.

The philosopher Jacquelyn Zita identifies a double bind in the norms of gynecology. On the one hand, it posits "relatively non-cyclic male physiology" as the measure of health, against which "female cyclicity is considered deviant" (1988, 81). This physiology is taken as the basis for sound psychological functioning. In 1974, Robert A. Kinch wrote in the *American Journal of Obstetrics and Gynecology*, "Premenstrual tension produces an oppressive, cyclic cloud which prevents women from functioning in a smooth, logical male fashion" (664). Not only does Kinch see male physiology as the measure of human health, but also he adds the irrelevant notion of logic, which he identifies as a male characteristic.

On the other hand, Zita continues, notions of female physiological health simultaneously assume a "continuously placid femininity," a state of sweetness, passivity, compliance: "The conditions associated with the premenstruum, such as irritability, aggression, violence, moodiness, are seen as 'deviant' [from the norms of passive femininity] . . . and apparently incapacitating (if 'disability' is defined as not accepting feminine roles or as disruptive to the linear organization of male social labor)" (81). Femininity becomes so elusive a quality as to disappear altogether when 95 percent of women are diagnosed with a syndrome defined by its absence. Yet gender role norms cannot be sacrificed, requiring the contruction of placid femininity as a *hormonal* norm. Given the idea of logic and calm as biologically male, no woman can satisfy this standard. Moreover, the medical gaze takes women's anger as evidence of female biological instability rather than a response to a world in which women are too often taken for granted, dismissed, and treated as less than full human beings. The moral and political aspects of women's interactions with others are thereby rendered meaningless, as if women had no interests at all.

Yet the gynecological norm that Zita identifies must be understood in moral and existential terms: femaleness as selflessness, existing for others, an erasure of subjectivity and personhood. This norm is expressed clearly when behaviors and processes in women are pathologized according to their inconvenience for others; that is, whether a trait is defined as "natural," "normal," or "functional" in women may be influenced by the needs or desires of men and children. Helen Roberts recounts the case of a woman who decided one morning never to do housework again, though she had not yet formulated other plans. When she informed her husband of this decision, he sent her to a general practitioner who diagnosed her as suffering from "Brainstorm" and recommended psychiatric treatment. After electroshock prescribed by the psychiatrist, she returned home and went back to doing housework (1985, 34–35).

Although this event took place over twenty-five years ago, the medical norm of female selflessness still persists when women are treated for PMS on the basis of their male partners' discomfort rather than their own. In the 1950s, physician Katharina Dalton was one of the originators of the term "premenstrual syndrome," from which she believed she herself suffered (Tavris 1992, 140; Sherwin 1992, 184). Dalton, like other medical authors sees a husband's complaint as sufficient reason to treat a woman for PMS.[12] Dalton sympathizes with the husband, terrified "when with little warning and no justification, his darling little love bird becomes an angry, argumentative, shouting, abusive bitch" (quoted in Zita 1988, 80).

Dalton goes as far as "blaming marital discord and family stresses on these periodic lapses in female placidity" (Zita 1988, 80), speculating: "How many wives batter their husbands during the premenstruum is unknown, nor do we know how often the husband is provoked beyond endurance and batters her" (quoted in Zita 1988, 80). There is clearly a relational and behavioral norm structuring this understanding of a female "syndrome": that is, women should strive for placidity rather than argue or express anger; women should avoid causing others discomfort, despite the costs to themselves. This norm pathologizes women's pursuit of their own interests in relationships with men while preserving the men's interests. A husband's denial of a wife's perceptions reemerges as concern for her health.

A diagnosis of PMS assumes inherent psychological disarray, regardless of the symptoms a woman identifies and reports or her view of them. Medical texts associate PMS, dysmenorrhea (menstrual pain), and menopause with psychological symptoms, recommending routine psychological screening for women reporting these physiological conditions (Rosenwaks, Benjamin, and Stone 1987, 92). *Novak's Textbook of Gynecology* notes that "suggestibility [to placebo] is a hallmark of the dysmenorrheic woman" (Jones, Wentz, and Burnett 1988, 246), and concludes that, in treating PMS, "little of permanent value can be expected from any therapeutic regimen without concomitant counseling, or perhaps psychotherapy" (259). While any chronic or recurring symptoms debilitating enough to require treatment are likely to have some psychological impact, it is by no means standard practice to address psychological issues in other such cases. That it is done selectively with "female problems" suggests the familiar historical perceptions of menstruation as a time of chaos and irrationality, of women as inherently emotional rather than logical.

Where interpersonal or other environmental issues are addressed, it is usually through individual psychological or familial characteristics (Jones, Wentz, and Burnett, 1988, 437–38), rather than in relation to a social context that devalues women and stigmatizes both menstruation and menopause as embarrassing, dirty, shameful, or disgusting. In short, the pathology, disturbance, lack, or inadequacy is understood to be rooted in women themselves, rather than in socially structured interactions of work, politics, interpersonal relations, and physiological processes. When the vast majority of *healthy* women are said to be afflicted with a "syndrome," for which treatment is required, it is femaleness itself that is pathologized. This contributes to women's alienation from our own bodies: imagine the experience of a teenage girl reading such statistics.

I do not mean to dismiss this syndrome as the product of an overheated medical imagination; many women do suffer from PMS and find some relief in various medical and self-help treatments. Yet on a broader social level, the diagnosis of PMS can rob women of coherence in the world. Interpreting women's perceptions on the basis of hormones undermines all women's social and political authority.

In practice, however, gynecology is problematic in different ways for different women. PMS borrows much of its cultural meaning from heterosexual marriage, and gynecological practice often treats this context as normative. Many lesbians and bisexual women fear coming out to their doctors because of heterosexist assumptions or outright discrimination.[13] One woman reports: "I went to the clinic hemorrhaging badly. The doctor, who knew I was a lesbian and not trying to get pregnant, insisted I was having a miscarriage" (Boston Women's Health Book Collective 1992, 190). Several studies document problems with care for lesbians, including one in which 72 percent of lesbians surveyed had experienced "negative reactions from health care providers concerning sexual orientation, including inappropriate treatment, refusal of care, and sexual harrassment" (O'Toole 1996, 145). It is no surprise, then, that as many as two-thirds of lesbians avoid Pap smears and other routine gynecological care (O'Toole 1996, 144).

Most participants in a study of women with disabilities sponsored by the National Institutes of Health also avoided gynecological care "out of fear" (Nosek 1996b, 25). Gynecologists are less likely to ask women with disabilities whether they are sexually active (Welner 1996, 81), and when they do, they are likely to assume heterosexuality (O'Toole 1996, 138). Women with disabilities need to have gynecological care integrated into rehabilitation settings, yet so far, integrated care is more likely to be available to men than to women (Waxman 1996). A number of the NIH study participants reported that their physicians "did not know how their disabilities affected sexual functioning, said nothing at all, or provided inaccurate information" (Nosek 1996b, 25).

HIV antibody–positive women also have difficulty getting the gynecological care they need; frequently it is not integrated into their primary care, despite the fact that primary care physicians are trained in gynecology. It should be integrated, however, writes nurse-practitioner and HIV primary care scholar Risa Denenberg, because many of the manifestations of HIV in women are gynecological, including altered menstrual cycles and "increased premenstrual symptoms" (1993, 42). Such integration is also important for the sake of continuity of care. Denenberg suggests that bias influences the gynecological neglect of women with HIV: "There may . . . be subconscious opinions that women with HIV infection become 'asexual' or that they should not have sex and therefore do not have the same concerns others have about menstruation, menopause, and sexuality" (43).

The issue here is not so much the complexity of accommodating needs based on sexual orientation, disability, or HIV status, although that is significant. Rather, the larger concern is how these problems manifest gynecology's model of the patient, which marginalizes or neglects some women's needs by defining others as "basic" or "normal," for example, by using prescription drugs and psychotherapy to prevent a woman's hormones from interfering with her femininity or creating discord in her marriage. It is striking that the boundaries between "normal" and "special" needs so often conform to social norms of femininity as selfless heterosexuality. Neither lesbians nor women with disabilities can be "real women," apparently, and thus their concerns are not central to gynecology. Their experiences show the desperate need for a material-semiotic medical theory and practice, one that attends to and accommodates the variations in women's circumstances, a need whose benefits are by no means limited to "special" groups.

Alice Dan, Linda Lewis, and the contributors to their collection *Menstrual Health in Women's Lives* (1992) exemplify such an approach, connecting women's perceptions and bodily experiences clearly to our life circumstances and social environments. Their account of women's health is conceptually richer than mainstream notions and far more hospitable to women's diverse interests. Menstruation and menopause are construed as "biocultural" phenomena, related to women's subjective experiences within a broader sociopolitical context. The authors emphasize "normal experience, the need to recognize interactions among many variables, and the challenge to negative connotations of menstruation," arguing that both "cultural stereotypes" and "clinical situations . . . tend to overemphasize problems in menstrual function" (4, 5). In their view, research must examine "social interaction, cultural perspectives, environmental changes, nutrition, family patterns, genetic factors, political actions, psychological

characteristics, and other sorts of information" along with "biological variables. . . . Thus, the study of menstrual health is necessarily multidisciplinary in nature" (5). The authors not only place women's subjective concerns at the center of analysis but also recognize women's agency in their
own health and in the world more broadly.

Feminist critics hold various positions on PMS: some see it as a "manu-
factured" diagnosis which stigmatizes femaleness, though it validates women's experiences (Tavris 1992, 134, 143). Others find it a useful diagnostic category and call for more precise research (Mitchell et al. 1992).
Debates over PMS treatments such as progesterone have "provided a plat-
form from which women have made themselves heard" (Lewis 1992, 68),
making it less likely that women's complaints will be neglected, as menstrual
pain often was in the past (Corea 1985, 267).

These critics tend to agree on the following points: women's experiences of menstruation have been and continue to be negatively affected
by medical and cultural stereotypes of menstruation, which have also stig-
matized women themselves;[14] research should attend to the sociocultural
context of menstruation, addressing it primarily as a healthful process, for
example, focusing on "premenstrual changes" rather than approaching it as
a "syndrome" foremost (Tavris 1992, 144); and treatment for menstrual
symptoms should be offered on the basis of women's self-defined needs
rather than others' complaints. I would add to this model the centrality of
inclusiveness, which is likely to enhance care for everyone.

Obstetrics

One might think that if female biology is conceptualized in mainly reproductive terms, with childbearing assigned normative value, then obstetrics might provide a welcome relief from gynecological negativism.[15] Unfortunately, this is not so. The professional process that began in an effort
to "search out and contain potential pathology" in childbirth (Arney 1982,
85) eventually led to defining birth as a crisis or emergency in all cases
rather than as a basically normal phenomenon, with exceptions.

With the use of modern technology, obstetrics developed a new relationship to the labor process which William Arney terms "monitoring,"

referring to the electronic fetal monitor but also more broadly to "a new mode of social control over childbirth" (1982, 100). Formerly, "the mother and fetus had to be treated as one unit while the fetus lay hidden inside the mother"; with the advent of electronic monitoring, however, practitioners could use instruments to apprehend the state of the fetus (Rothman 1989, 157). They could then distinguish sharply between the perceived needs of woman and fetus, and thus choose between them. This made it possible to prioritize the fetus, now understood as separate and vulnerable, in need of medical rather than maternal protection, consisting of an array of interventions affecting fetus and woman both. Arney writes, "After the monitoring concept was in place, obstetrics did not need to confine itself to the abnormal or potentially pathological birth; every birth became subject to its gaze" (100).

The array of interventions includes various techniques that can be life-saving in certain kinds of crises (Arms 1977, 64): electronic fetal monitoring, the artificial rupture of amniotic membranes to stimulate labor, anesthesia (which may be administered or denied contrary to the woman's preference), forceps delivery, and episiotomy or incision, as well as lithotomy (keeping the woman supine on a table throughout labor). The analyses of journalist and patient advocate Suzanne Arms (1977) and of Doris Haire (1972), a medical sociologist with an honorary doctorate in medical science, demonstrate that each intervention performed—all of which are common, some routine—will usually entail the need for further interventions, creating the opportunity for a variety of complications to arise which affect both woman and infant. Each procedure, though invaluable in emergencies, is also associated in various ways with increased discomfort and risk for woman, infant, or both, yet has not been established as medically necessary *except* in unusual cases—which may seem more prevalent than they would otherwise, given that performing any one intervention is likely to create the very complications that call for others in turn.

The supine position, for example, adversely affects a woman's blood pressure and cardiac functioning, with the risk of decreasing the fetal oxygen supply. It can also weaken contractions and undermine her ability to push by interfering with the effects of gravity. Episiotomies and forceps deliveries are more likely than when a woman is fully or partially upright. Even the positioning of her feet in stirrups increases pressure on her perineum, and thus the likelihood of an episiotomy. Moreover, her feet are not adequately separated to allow for natural expulsion (Arms 1977, 102–4). Finally, the psychological effects of this position should not be underestimated, as it fosters a sense of vulnerability and even humiliation.

Obstetric femininity is quite congruent with that of gynecology. Anne Seiden argues that standard medicalized childbirth requires or assumes behavior based on "the so-called feminine personality," such as "passivity, dependence, ineptness, emotional lability, and sexual inhibition" (1978, 98). These qualities are "so exactly opposite to the requirements of good birth experience and good motherhood that one suspects that they are desired because of a poorly worked-through fear of mature women" (98). Perhaps this is the same fear reflected in the gynecology text's vocabulary of failing, exhausted, and disturbed menopausal processes.

It is striking that a birthing practice which has so little to recommend it from a woman's point of view could have become standardized. Many commentators have noted that the lithotomy position was clearly invented for the convenience of the physician at the expense of the birthing woman. Lithotomy, and the practice of electronic fetal monitoring which it supports, are equally determined by the episteme of the clinic, the scale of the gaze. Since Doris Haire's and Suzanne Arms's critiques of medicalized childbirth appeared in the early 1970s, medicalized childbirth has changed in many ways—a shift that is likely due as much to a competitive market which requires attending to women's consumer demands as it is to "advances" in medical understandings, although market-sensitive changes tend to be explained on grounds of the latter. Yet what has not changed is the underlying principle that structures medical knowledge in opposition to women's subjective experiences.

A number of established interests converge in the standardization of various medical interventions. The medical sociologist William Arney argues that the routineness of lithotomy and other such practices is due as much to historical and political developments in the status of the profession as to "medical" reasons (1982, 64–69). Moreover, the medical profession has strong financial ties to pharmaceutical companies and other medical industries, with the American Medical Association (AMA) receiving a significant portion of its yearly income from pharmaceutical advertising revenue (Arms 1977, 93).

According to the philosopher Susan Sherwin, routinizing interventions useful in emergencies "increas[es] medical control over the various aspects of women's reproductive lives. . . . Medically supervised pregnancies and hospital births are demanded of everyone; women who fail to comply may be subject to criminal prosecution for endangering the health of the fetus. . . . [D]octors decide when to use cesarean sections and are even prepared to get court orders to perform them if the pregnant woman does not 'consent'" (1992, 127–28). Such control is another instance of medicine prescribing selflessness for women, this time negating women's agency by promoting medical expertise as the only relevant criterion for decision making.

Obstetrics defines legitimate needs and interests as those that are unequivocally medical, separates the interests of fetuses and infants from those of women, and then categorizes women's interests as patients (including social and emotional needs of women and their families) as whims, frivolous or even selfish choices most likely conflicting with infants' needs. Medical literature has been known to refer to the pregnant woman as "the route to the fetus" (Overall 1987, 90), conceptualizing the relation between woman and fetus adversarially, their needs inherently in conflict. The infant becomes the primary patient because of greater dependency and therefore greater need. An intervention for the infant's benefit, whether the woman agrees to it or not, may be "seen as a *medical* decision rather than a moral or ethical one," as if women had no interests to be considered (Overall 1987, 94).

Although planned home births are not inherently dangerous, women who seek to integrate such values into giving birth as the physical and emotional comfort of remaining at home with family and friends are accused of risking their infants' lives, selfishly choosing their own well-being over that of their infants. Defining childbirth as a medical event per se automatically renders important human concerns frivolous or incidental at best, negligent at worst (Overall 1987, 101).

Moreover, not all events involving some degree of risk are likely to be treated as medical in nature. The sociologist Barbara Katz Rothman argues that "socially acceptable risks" in pregnancy and birth are those that involve "following the doctor's orders"; even practices that may be quite risky (for example, taking dangerous drugs during pregnancy such as diet pills or the synthetic hormone DES, later found to be carcinogenic) are socially approved when consistent with current medical standards (1982, 16–17).

Women of color are especially likely to be treated as inherently selfish, incapable of giving the proper weight to fetal interests. Angela Davis identifies "contradictions in the ideology of motherhood" which they face: "(1) criticism of young black mothers, (2) sterilization based on race and class, and (3) separation of incarcerated mothers from their children" (1994, 47). African American women are much more likely than others to be reported or convicted for drug use in pregnancy, a practice that discourages them from seeking prenatal care or drug treatment for fear of being arrested (Roberts 1994, 126–29). There are also racial disparities in forced medical treatment such as court-ordered cesareans (Roberts 1994, 132–34).

Similar problems can be seen in the situation of HIV-positive pregnant women. Seventy-five percent of women with AIDS are women of color (Shaw 1997). Although the number of infants contracting HIV from mothers has declined markedly in recent years ("Estimated Number" 1997), public efforts to control AIDS have centered on mandatory testing of newborns.[16] Such a policy would identify infants who would benefit from treatment, yet would fail to prevent HIV transmission, while reinforcing notions of pregnancy and birth as an adversarial conflict between woman and fetus. This is another instance in the often-noted tendency to treat women as "vessels and vectors" of AIDS transmission, rather than addressing the needs of women themselves.[17] A medically and morally beneficial alternative to mandatory testing of newborns would be to ensure that adequate prenatal care and HIV counseling and treatment are available to *all* women. Yet while universal health care is perceived as politically unthinkable, medical policing is widely accepted. Medical supervision thus becomes the socially sanctioned *moral* supervision of a group of people already perceived as untrustworthy on the basis of race, class, and gender.

In pathologizing "normal" childbirth, the health care system still privileges some women at the expense of others. Even though these women — white, middle class, able-bodied, young (but not too young), heterosexual, married, HIV negative — face paternalism, at least medicine grants them a reproductive identity, albeit a minimized one. The women who do not fit obstetrics' restrictive norms of patienthood experience worse than paternalism: neglect, coercion, and criminalization.

Whether in socially approved childbirth, or in births perceived as even more dangerous because unacceptable in some way, defining childbirth as an event of inherent medical risk removes health from the context of human life. Giving birth, writes Christine Overall, is "a transitional episode in a woman's life, a transformative event that . . . should not be abstracted from other life experiences and treated as an isolated medical event" (1987, 195). Doing so "alienates women from their own reproductive experiences," says Susan Sherwin (1992, 128), and diminishes a woman's sense of self, as Ann Oakley's sociology of childbirth demonstrates. Her study finds a significant correlation between a high degree of intervention in the birth process and "negative maternal outcome," including postpartum depression (1980). These findings testify to the importance of fostering women's sense of competence or efficacy through full participation in the decision making and the physical processes of childbirth.[18]

This need is clearly salient around the event of giving birth, which is not only a tremendous physiological upheaval but a highly significant life transition as well. Standard obstetric care fails to accommodate these values and needs; in fact, it tends to oppose them. Efficacy also applies to this chapter's previous examples. Menstrual health is a life experience which can reflect and reinforce a woman's sense of herself. Women need to be able to trust our own perceptions of our bodies and our experiences, a goal that gynecological theory and practice should respect and support. Rapists and batterers assault women's sense of competence and efficacy along with our bodies, and this sense can be undermined further by medical care after an assault. Yet this confidence in one's own powers and worth is essential for a woman to leave a batterer and make a new life, or regain a sense of safety and control in the world again.

In a deep sense, the medical norm of selflessness, as I have argued at various points in this chapter, involves an existential erasure of women's subjectivities. Medicine regulates many of the life experiences of women. It enforces its own definitions of reality over women's perceptions, often pursuing its goals at the expense of women's, or shaping women's goals to fit its own. Survivors of domestic violence may be treated for their physical injuries, while perhaps deeper psychological injuries are ignored—invisible to the clinical gaze, or outside its bounds—as if these subjective states of suffering, the damage to women's self-esteem and sense of agency, were insignificant. Medicine imposes its own psychological norms on women, as if there were one correct and healthy response to a given situation rather than a variety. In some of the situations I have discussed, medical practice is more concerned with a woman's conformity to preconceived notions of appropriate behavior or emotional state than with her subjective experience. This explains the ironic situation of medical theory ignoring the psychological injuries of battery while remaining preoccupied with the perceived emotionality of premenstrual and menopausal women.

Recall the earlier discussion of "the scale of the gaze," Foucault's metaphor for the epistemic principle of modern medicine. Knowledge is valued for its precise quantifiability, its detachment, understood to render it pure and objective, untainted by the body or the idiosyncrasy of individual consciousness. This epistemic norm clearly does not accommodate the subjectivities of laypersons or professionals—and these experiential aspects of health and illness must be included in the construction of knowledge. Compare the data produced by electronic fetal monitoring to the information gained by midwives empirically, intuitively, and from their own subjective states as well as those of laboring women—two quite distinct modes of knowledge, one of which has lost, and one of which has gained, cultural authority.[19]

Even more clearly than midwifery, however, the feminist critical perspectives discussed in this chapter exemplify this point, and show the distinct advantages as well of a medical perspective that incorporates egalitarian norms. The feminist authors I have cited analyze medicine from their concrete social locations as women, as feminists, and as researchers and practitioners who integrate these values into their work. Thus, their contributions depend as much on the goals and methods of the women's movement as they do on the goals and methods of their academic and professional disciplines. As activists they seek two closely connected ends: to transform material conditions, and to give women a greater voice in the social definition of reality.

Yet the modern medical paradigm—the scale of the gaze, or the Flexnerian model defended by Seldin—defines such moral commitments as the corruption of pure science with alien values. Are we therefore to reject the medical gaze, to refuse, for example, the diagnostic arsenal of X rays, endoscopes, ultrasound, and magnetic resonance imaging? Some critics may indeed reject the institution of medicine altogether, or nearly so,[20] but this is not my position. Instead I argue that the unnecessarily and inappropriately reductionistic scale of the gaze must give way to another model, one that includes the inherent moral, social, and political aspects of the embodied human concerns in medicine.

❦

2

Physician, Queer Thyself: Homophobia, Erotophobia, and Medicine

Lesbians, gay men, and bisexuals are not easily seduced by the romantic myth of modern medicine as the entirely benevolent, healing face of technology. Many participants in the gay liberation movement perceive medicine as contributing to their diminished status owing to the privileged form of moral—hence political—authority which it wields. Despite the fact that this cultural authority resides largely in the presumed objectivity of medical science, value judgments against members of oppressed groups continue to be expressed in the practice of medicine as well as in the broader social uses of medical discourse. For example, as Timothy F. Murphy (1992) points out, certain formal medical claims about homoeroticism may have been retracted, yet continued interest in practices such as conversion therapy suggests that judgments of the inferiority of homoeroticism can still be found in medicine.

I argue in this chapter that medicine promotes homophobia through its implicit moral authority, its power to shape cultural perceptions of groups and categories of people, and that it thereby perpetuates the oppression of a social group whose members already face other widespread harms.[1] While bioethics has begun to address some aspects of medical homophobia, what has not been adequately explored is the larger framework of medicine's cultural status. A material-semiotic analysis of HIV as a context of homophobia, which interacts with other oppressive beliefs and practices, is essential

43

to this project. I begin by reviewing the medicalization of homosexuality, turn to heterosexism and homophobia in HIV medicine, then explore their intersection with another social-medical norm, "erotophobia" (Patton 1985). Cultural erotophobia goes beyond fear and hatred of homosexuality, encompassing other aspects of sexuality which are considered deviant, yet its hierarchical norms help to explain the existence and persistence of homophobia in particular.

I broaden the scope of analysis in this way in order to illuminate significant continuities in the cultural treatment of both "female sexuality" (constructed as heterosexual) and lesbian, bisexual, and gay male sexuality. Drawing on the previous chapter, I argue that, despite the differences in the medicalization of "women's" sexuality and that of "gay" sexuality, they share important commonalities nonetheless which are seldom addressed in bioethics or social and political philosophy.[2] These continuities must be recognized in the moral evaluation of the medicine of sexuality, social difference, and HIV. Furthermore, the medicalization of deviant or "queer" sexuality, like that of femaleness, indicates the inadequacy of typical conceptions of the principle of objectivity, which is a vital concern for bioethics.

The Medicalization of Homosexuality

Given how AIDS was first conceptualized in Western industrialized countries as a "gay disease," it is important to situate the epidemic in the historical context of the medicalization of homosexuality itself. Jeffrey Weeks writes that in the late nineteenth century, "medicine was replacing the Church as the moulder of public opinion," substituting "the new sanctions of madness, moral insanity, sickness and disease" for the old category of sin (1977, 23). In the process, the concept of "moral contagion" was applied to homosexuality, with lesbianism perceived as "a congenital disease," like male homosexuality, yet "the lesser crime" of the two (Phelan 1989, 25). The new science of sexology searched for a physiological or genetic understanding of homosexuality, motivated in part because new criminal codes required a definitive answer as to whether "deviant" individuals were responsible for their sexual acts. If homosexuality was a congenital phenomenon, then homosexuals should not be subjected to the judgment of the court. If, however, homosexuality was acquired, then homosexuals were criminals who bore full legal and moral responsibility for their sexual acts, and should be judged as such.

Although medical discourse surely influenced the eventual trend toward decriminalization in Britain and the United States, Weeks illuminates the more subtle power dynamics at work, attributing the eventual success of the disease model of homosexuality largely to its compatibility with middle-class norms: how else to explain the violation of decency and respectability, the perversions of "otherwise ordinary middle-class people," except by madness (28)? Of course, there was a serious cost to this new understanding of homosexuality as an illness: it entailed treating homosexuals not only with pity but with aggressive medicine as well—drugs, castration, hypnotherapy, psychoanalysis, aversion therapy—a clear and direct instance of medicine as a form of social control. While the medical model was hotly contested for many years by those who sought to punish homosexuals for crimes against nature, it nevertheless managed to gain such influence that "by 1965, 93 percent of those polled in an opinion poll saw homosexuality as a form of illness requiring medical treatment" (Weeks 1977, 30).

It is important to understand what was at stake in this process. Jonathan Katz identifies the professional and class interests of doctors in the medicalization of homosexuality:

> The historical change in the conception of homosexuality from sin to crime to sickness is intimately associated with the rise to power of a class of petit bourgeois medical professionals, a group of individual medical entrepreneurs, whose stock in trade is their alleged "expert" understanding of homosexuality, a special interest group whose facade of scientific objectivity covers their own emotional, economic, and career investments in their status as such authorities. (1976, 199)

These class interests do not tell the whole story, however. Also at stake was the status of medical discourse, its hegemonic power to define reality. "Homosexuality" presented an opportunity for the medical profession to define the terms of an important social debate and thus advance its claim that medical representations of social phenomena expressed fundamental truths of nature.

In an important sense, medicine can be said to have invented the figure of the homosexual. Although legal prohibitions of homosexual acts abounded for centuries before the science of sexology existed, "there was no concept of the homosexual in law, and homosexuality was regarded not as a particular attribute of a certain type of person but as a potential in all sinful creatures" (Weeks 1977, 12).[3] Thus medicine constituted homosexuals as such through its powers of definition, providing a new sense of self, released from the bonds of sin into another kind of shame: "If the law and its associated penalties made homosexuals into outsiders, and religion gave them a high sense of guilt, medicine and science gave them a deep sense of inferiority and inadequacy" (Weeks 1977, 31).

This shame continued to manifest itself throughout the twentieth century. A sense of congenitality may lift the burden of responsibility yet replace it with the stigma of deviance and abnormality. Literary works such as James Baldwin's *Just above My Head* (1978), Barbara Deming's *A Humming under My Feet* (1985), and Martin Duberman's *Cures* (1991) tell movingly of the struggles of lesbians, bisexuals, and gay men to accept themselves in the 1950s and 1960s. The pain of psychiatric stigmatizing is a frequent theme in works dealing with this era. Deming writes of traveling in Europe and meeting a gay man also from the United States:

> He had a friend back home who had told him he was sick and should see a psychiatrist. But the day after he told him this he'd gone not to the psychiatrist but to a travel agency. He'd flown away here. . . . If his friend thought he was sick because he was a homosexual, that was nonsense, I assured him (as I had learned to assure myself). . . . He sat considering my words. And then—I can remember the look still—he glanced down at himself, down at the full length of his graceful body, and an expression of utter disgust twisted his face. He whispered, "I wish this body didn't exist." He whispered, "I wish it weren't here." Then he turned to me with a beseeching look, as though I could somehow unwish his wish. (135)

Medicine may exonerate the individual from the blame attached to sin and vice, but in its place can leave a profound self-hatred and sense of annihilation, including a deep alienation from the body. Some aspects of PMS medicine undermine women's sense of self by attributing their subjective emotional states to physiological disturbances perceived as virtually synonymous with femaleness (see Chapter 1). In this case, the pathologizing of homoerotic desire becomes a taboo against embracing, even accepting, the gay, lesbian, or bisexual self. This also creates another kind of selflessness, blocking the possibility of articulating one's interests related to homoerotic desire, identity, and practice. Pathology presupposes that one's interests consist of cure where possible, otherwise managing symptoms or rehabilitation—which in this case can only result in alienation from one's sexuality and thus self-devaluation.

Not only does pathologization militate against gay self-acceptance, but also it prescribes a certain set of social relations. Shane Phelan argues that medicalization treats "issues of sexuality" as "matters of health, and thus as individual in nature . . . [their] social unacceptability . . . assumed; it is the 'disease' or 'character disorder' that needs explanation and treatment, not the social structure or attitudes" (1989, 26). Thus, homosexuality is cast not as a social identity but as a malady which befalls some unfortunate individuals, absolving heterosexuals of the moral responsibility to account for their disapproval and differential treatment of lesbians, gay men, and bisexuals.

In summary, while the disease model of homosexuality tended to subvert outright moral blame for homoerotic acts and desires, it did not release lesbians, gay men, and bisexuals into an era of unambiguous enlightenment. Instead, it replaced moral shame with the shame of biological inferiority or deviance. It also reinforced both the middle-class norms of (heterosexual) respectability and the moral authority of medicine, themes that persist in the medicalization of AIDS.

It is useful at this point to distinguish certain aspects of the term medicine which, until now, I have not separated. The following are four conceptually distinct aspects of medicine, though they may overlap in practice:

1. The practices of individual providers and the rules and systems of specific medical institutions.

2. Medical discourse as it is presented to laypersons in mainstream media and filtered through popular culture; medical information as used in various nonmedical contexts.

3. Biomedical theory and specific conceptualizations of organs, systems, processes, diseases, and pathologies; recognized standards of care; "expert" medical discourse on its own terms.

4. Medicine as cultural myth, based in large part on its actual or perceived relation to science, which is accorded the epistemic status of indisputable Truth. (As a character exhorted in *Flatliners,* a 1990 horror
movie, "Philosophy has failed. Religion has failed. Now it's up to physical
science!")

A vital recognition of feminists and AIDS activists is that the first three
aspects of medicine are frequently mediated through ideologies of gender,
sexual orientation, and other social categories. The fourth helps to justify
and support these ideologies manifested in the representations and practices of the first three.

Each of these facets of medicine has profound political implications on
its own; together they constitute an even more significant manifestation of
power. Particular instances of the first two elements, while they may be
extremely influential, are nevertheless relatively easy to call into question.
For example, medical ethicists and consumer activists have had great success in illuminating, if not eradicating, problems in the traditional doctor-
patient relationship. As for the variety of medical information presented in
the mass media, it is understood by its very nature to be a kind of watered-
down, roughly schematic representation of "the facts themselves," which
are perceived as too complicated for laypersons to grasp. Thus the third
level enjoys a greater status—that of factuality—for this very reason, despite the frequent revision of many individual concepts (such as the defeat
of the proto-gynecological dogma that the study of Latin caused the ova-
ries of young girls to wither away). Finally, it is the cultural power of medicine as myth, as expression of a society's fundamental needs, goals, and values, which has the most unshakable status, owing to its association with the
supposed purity and objective detachment of science "itself."

I turn now to examples of homophobic concepts and practices at each of
these levels.

Practices of Providers and Institutions

Since the early 1990s, problems of access, medical prejudice and incompe-
tence, and interference with the support of partners and friends have been
documented in the context of HIV. Many providers demonstrate reluc-

tance or outright refusal to treat persons who are HIV positive. In Minnesota, for example, despite the existence of a Human Rights Act which outlaws discrimination on the basis of disability or sexual orientation, a Health Department study found that "21 percent of 241 HIV-infected respondents could not find a dentist willing to treat them" ("Minnesota Dentist" 1992). This is not a purely midwestern phenomenon: 48 percent of physicians responding to a 1992 Los Angeles County survey refused to treat HIV-positive patients ("Doctors Balk" 1992). Many rural AIDS patients must struggle to find doctors who will treat them (Booth 1993), and "reports of emergency service workers who refuse to treat or transport AIDS patients have surfaced throughout the country, even in large metropolitan areas such as New York" (Chibbaro 1994, 29). And in a survey of over 1,800 AIDS patients in the United States, "more than 36 percent reported acts of discrimination when receiving health care" ("Survey Reveals Abuse" 1992, A22).

General medical homophobia undoubtedly exerts a strong influence in HIV medicine, as broader medical contexts suggest. A review of nine studies from 1970 to 1990 reports widespread perceptions among physicians that medical schools should not teach lesbian health issues, and that "lesbians themselves should not be allowed as medical students or teachers" (Plumb 1996, 55). Ninety percent of alternative insemination providers will not offer the procedure to lesbians or other unmarried women (Zarembka 1996, 43). In 1991 the *Journal of the American Medical Association* reported, "Thirty-five percent of 1,121 physicians questioned . . . agreed that 'homosexuality is a threat to many of our institutions.' The survey also found that 68 percent of the physicians felt ethically bound to treat AIDS patients, but 17 percent did not" ("Survey Reveals Doctors" 1991).

Charles Bosk and Joel Frader cite a medical ethics discussion group in a medical school that does not permit students to "refuse to care for HIV-positive patients. The policy infuriates many students. . . . They said such rules have no place in medicine. Doctors, they believe, should have as much freedom as lawyers, accountants, executives, or others to accept or reject 'clients' or 'customers'" (1991, 159). Bosk and Frader note that many doctors and medical students openly express their resentment of "guilty" patients.

Unwillingness to treat can in many cases be directly attributed to bias.

Rose Weitz cites studies which "have found that up to 76 percent of doctors would prefer not to treat persons with HIV disease because they either fear infection or believe such persons do not deserve their services" (1991, 80). She notes, "Another study concluded that nursing, medical, and chiropractic students . . . all considered persons with AIDS less competent and less morally worthy than persons with cancer, diabetes, or heart disease" (25), a particularly disturbing discrepancy, given that our society attributes a high degree of personal responsibility for the latter diseases because of their association with lifestyle. Similarly, Michael D. Quam reports differences between nurses' treatment of people with AIDS whom they consider "innocent victims" and those they perceive as guilty (1990, 37). Weitz interviewed people with AIDS whose treatment conveyed these attitudes:

> Some doctors . . . make their ignorance and prejudice immediately known . . . by adopting unnecessary precautions against contagion such as donning gowns and masks, informing people who are infected with HIV but have yet to develop any opportunistic infections that they will die within a few months, speaking rudely or abruptly, and [as late as 1989] warning persons with HIV disease that they can infect their families if they hug them, cook their meals, or wash their clothes. (64)

The rules and habits of medical institutions intersect with the legal status of gays and lesbians to limit their rights when a partner or other "chosen family" member (Weston 1991) is hospitalized with AIDS. Jeffrey Levi, former executive director of the National Gay and Lesbian Task Force, states: "The legal system . . . does not recognize the family relationships that gays and lesbians form. Gay lovers have no legal standing—whether in seeking spousal benefits or in simpler issues like visitation rights at hospitals" (1986, 180). In a front-page *Washington Post* story on the status of lesbians and gay men, a woman tells of trying to visit her partner hospitalized with pneumonia, only to be "stopped by hospital rules allowing only a spouse or relative to enter" (Sanchez and Morin 1993). Hospitals may deny gay men and lesbians visitation by lovers, friends, and representatives of gay and lesbian service agencies, all of whom often function as family (Blumenfeld and Raymond 1988, 257–58; Keen 1996; Patton 1985, 69–70; Plumb 1996).

The case of Sharon Kowalski, who suffered brain damage and partial paralysis in an accident, and her partner, Karen Thompson, helped to bring this issue to public attention. Kowalski's parents obtained guardianship and denied Thompson visitation rights or any other role in Kowalski's care, forcing Thompson to endure a lengthy legal battle to be with her partner and support her recovery (Blumenfeld and Raymond 1988, 257–58). The HIV epidemic drastically increased the number of people facing this problem. As a result, the PWA (People with AIDS) Coalition's "Patient's Bill of Rights" affirms "the right to the choice of 'immediate family member' status for those the patient may designate" ("PWA Coalition Portfolio" 1988, 160).

Undoubtedly, many people with AIDS have received compassionate and competent care. Many others, however, have faced serious obstacles as a result of providers' unwillingness to treat them, the prejudice and ignorance of providers, and the failure of others to recognize chosen family members' role in their care. In the context of HIV, this burden is differentially imposed on gay and bisexual men (although it also affects others insofar as they are perceived as having a "gay disease"). It affects prognosis if needed care is delayed as a result, and imposes isolation as well as practical difficulties if partners and friends are shut out of their roles. The devastation of disease can only be magnified by the devastation of medical fears, callousness, and indifference, which in turn reinforce other oppressive practices and exacerbate the loss of agency and control which may be imposed by illness itself. This cumulative burden faced by gay and bisexual men with AIDS is deeply unjust. Although it has often been addressed by medical ethicists and in the popular press, the bioethical concerns related to HIV do not stop here by any means, as my survey of other aspects of medicine indicates.

Medical Information in Mass Media and Popular Culture

Oppressive influences can readily be detected in popular health and medical discourse. What is presented as medical advice in these domains may actually be based on moralistic assumptions which are neither made explicit nor defended, a point that is particularly salient with respect to AIDS.

Cultural conservatives' discussions of the epidemic frequently conflate the language of medical pathology with the moral language of sin and retribution, lending a scientific air to moral and political pronouncements. A right-wing organization in Texas, seeking to reinstate an anti-sodomy law which had been declared unconstitutional in that state, invoked the moral and rhetorical authority of medicine by calling itself "Dallas Doctors against AIDS" (Altman 1987, 69). Conservatives have gone so far as to claim medical grounds for the censorship of certain artworks, such as the "link between art and disease . . . drawn by the president of the Massachusetts chapter of Morality in Media, who was reported to have said, 'People looking at these kinds of pictures become addicts and spread AIDS'" (Eberly 1992, 207). Similarly, Senator Jesse Helms claimed that the National Endowment for the Arts would "promote" homosexuality and thus foster HIV transmission by supporting art with gay or lesbian themes or sexual content (Carter 1992, 12).[4]

It is no surprise that conservatives already appalled by the movement whose theme was "gay pride" would find the AIDS epidemic reason to condemn not just sexual practices associated with gay men but gay identity itself. For example, conservative commentator Gene Antonio invokes scientific authority in defense of homophobia: "Homosexuality per se must be taught as an unhealthy, unsafe and lethal sexual alternative. 'It's a very major risk to enter these communities,' warns June Osborn, Dean of Public Health at the University of Michigan and a professor of epidemiology. 'So tell the fifteen or sixteen-year-old kid who's going to declare his same-sex preference that there's a serious chance of infection that can truly be a matter of life and death' (1988, 133). Antonio conflates "entering a community" and "declaring a preference" with unsafe sexual practices, assigning moral blame to all of these. His emphasis on the deadliness of homosexuality underscores the danger of gay identity and desire, even as it obscures the fact that it is specific practices, by no means exclusive to those who identify as gay nor inclusive of all who do, which put one at risk of HIV transmission—practices, moreover, that are not biologically determined by ineluctable sexual essences but are social creations.

When Antonio quotes June Osborn, he chooses to omit a crucial part of her original statement, which appears in an article by John Langone (1985). She continues: "The false hope of a vaccine or a cure prevents people from examining their sexual options. False hopes keep people from having to face up to the fact that prevention is the most rational thing, and it is possible—not easy, but possible" (53). Unhealthy, unsafe, lethal; options, rational, prevention, possible. The tone has changed from that of Antonio's moral apocalypse to a call for prudence—a significant difference. Invoking the scientific verification lent by the epidemiologist's professional stature, Antonio implies that responsibility in sexual choices is a contradiction in terms for gay men; yet such responsibility is exactly what the omitted portion of Osborn's statement emphasizes. Moreover, Osborn undercuts an unreflective faith in medicine by emphasizing responsible decision making; she suggests that people must negotiate between options rather than submit to a given moral-medical imperative.

An important question at this juncture is whether conservative attitudes toward homoeroticism are oppressive yet remediable by increased medical sophistication. After all, one may object, medicine "itself" is in no way implicated by political (mis)uses of medical information. Moreover, Osborn's brief comment is not reducible to political diatribe and even gives the useful, if basic, advice to weigh one's options; it does not offer plain condemnation. It is not terribly surprising that right-wing condemnations of gay sexual identity and of people with AIDS invoke medical authority. Yet mainstream media representations of AIDS, as well as medical concepts— ostensibly politically neutral or value-free—also tacitly reproduce these same right-wing attitudes (as I argue in the next section). Thus popular and expert medical discourses not only are frequently difficult to separate but are also susceptible to ideological influence and available for tacit political service.

A different kind of problem which can be associated with the second aspect of medicine is the intersection of homophobia with issues of racism and ethnocentrism in the presentation of risk-reduction information. Many analysts have noted the failure of approaches that implicitly assume a white middle-class perspective. For example, a psychotherapeutic group model may try to foster safer sex practices by having participants discuss their feelings about their sexuality and about changing their sexual practices. Such an approach may be useful for white middle-class people, but in many other cultural settings there may be resistance to discussing sexuality openly, or even to psychotherapy in its middle-class manifestations.

Moreover, members of a racially oppressed group may see little reason to trust speakers who are racially and economically privileged, and may also feel a strong need to dissociate themselves from the "gay plague," or simply from the general stigma attached to AIDS. The experience of racial denigration and the need to preserve community ties may make it very difficult to undertake HIV prevention. According to Dooley Worth's study of two New York City AIDS prevention programs, "women who live in minority communities are marked as being at risk or having AIDS merely by asking a question about it. As a result, many women are afraid to even ask for information on AIDS because it will stigmatize them" (1989, 306). AIDS educators concerned with this issue advocate a variety of techniques involving the resources of particular communities, such as integrating AIDS information into neighborhood and organized group activities (Ports 1990, 111).

How deep are these problems in medical information as it is transmitted through popular channels? One may argue that medicine should not be used to lend rhetorical/moral weight to nonmedical judgments, yet feel that the problem here is not with "medicine" itself but with its rhetorical uses for ideological purposes. And the clear solution to this problem is not somehow to *transcend* the authority of medicine but in fact to wield that authority in the service of accuracy, for example, using medical information to establish the counterproductiveness of mandatory HIV screening of various groups, or other such restrictions. Regarding the intersections of racism and ethnocentrism with homophobia in HIV education, some would respond that the information "itself" is no less valuable, even though it may require adjustments in cultural relevance and clarity—a problem of rhetoric, one might say, but not of medicine.

My claim, however, is that separating medical pronouncements into "content" and "rhetoric" is not so simple, given that language does not passively "represent" ideas themselves but rather structures content fundamentally. This is one of the crucial insights of a material-semiotic analysis. Furthermore, even if such a separation were possible, the cultural authority of medicine grounds not only the "content" of information but also its use in specific contexts. By definition, the "rhetorical modifications" necessary to make health information culturally relevant to specific groups are constructed as foreign, extrinsic to the "facts," which are understood as existing outside any human social context rather than interwoven into it. At the same time, the white middle-class perspective from which those "facts" were initially conceptualized, and then reformulated for laypersons, is thereby validated as the medical view from nowhere. Employing medical discourse in social policy struggles is strategically necessary and practically unavoidable. Yet the underlying problem of medicine's unchallenged authority as the fundamental truth of human existence still remains.

Biomedical Theory and Specific Conceptualizations

I have suggested that popular and expert medical discourses are connected in the following way: scientific data are used to shore up moral and political judgments, which are then presented in the form of medical information for the masses. Pathologization, however, takes forms that are *simultaneously* medical and moral. Homophobia significantly influences many scientific conceptualizations of HIV transmission. Furthermore, even in the absence of overtly homophobic attitudes on the part of researchers, the marginalized status of lesbians, gays, and bisexuals means that there is already a lack of knowledge about gay sexuality, frequently so much so that researchers are not aware that information may be incomplete or inaccurate. This situation further complicates the difficult project of obtaining accurate HIV transmission information, and functions to reinforce homophobia and gay oppression by failing to challenge "medical" claims that are actually based on tacit moral assumptions.

A construction of difference as Otherness shapes information regarding the transmission of HIV (Byron 1991; Treichler 1988a, b; Watney 1989). Not only do such perceptions of difference affect the way the "facts" are presented, but they also affect the way the "facts" are *conceptualized*. In the early years of the epidemic, for example, transmission information focused on identities and "risk groups" rather than practices, imposing a dichotomy between a riskless Us and a jeopardized Them. Jan Zita Grover (1988), Cindy Patton (1985, 1990), Paula Treichler (1988a, b), Simon Watney (1989), and others have rightly noted that the term "general population," often used in measuring the significance of the epidemic, is implicitly white, middle-class, and heterosexual, an identity perceived not as a social creation but as codified somehow in nature itself, certified as safe and natural because outside so-called risk groups.

In this light, AIDS can be understood as a social crisis not only in the obvious epidemiological sense but also in terms of the moral and political contradictions it reveals. Homoeroticism is perceived as impossible—or possible only in the realm of the Other. In ordinary times, as opposed to crises, social boundaries are both invisible and unconscious; experienced as impermeable, inevitable, a fact of nature. Yet viruses fail to heed a society's doctrines about gender and sexual orientation—who is "supposed" to get sick and who is not.

Even such disparate icons of heterosexual masculinity as actor Rock Hudson, basketball star Earvin(Magic) Johnson, and rapper Eazy E are not immune. AIDS exposes their status as *representations* of masculinity rather than paradigmatic instances of "the real thing," namely, heterosexual masculinity as a fundamental truth of nature. Their respective associations with AIDS call into question the very existence of that paradigm—the real man, protected by nature, which made him as he is—raising anxieties that "anyone" (read any man) is susceptible. Inevitably, such fears lead to reinforced boundaries of race, class, gender, and sexuality: real straight men versus those (homosexuals) who only play them on screen, respectable (white) family men versus "promiscuous" (black) sports stars, and upstanding (white) protectors of women versus out-of-control (black) "gangsters." In the process, myths of gay male perversion (Mohr 1998), bisexual male duplicity (White 1996), and black male predatory sexuality (hooks 1992, 87–113) take on new life.

The epidemic, then, unsettles social boundaries which provide those who are privileged with a sense of security. This transgression is then cast as both the cause and the sign of inevitable social, psychological, and medical havoc. First perceived as a gay phenomenon, HIV has been discussed and represented in terms of its "spread," "containment," and "saturation," as if it had "natural" limits which are in danger of violation (Grover 1988; Treichler 1988b, 65–66). Such notions frequently result in calls to reinforce social boundaries through means such as immigration controls and restrictions on homosexual content in goverment-funded art and educational materials.[5]

Many constructions of the "facts" of transmission have involved the pathologization of gay male sexuality in the guise of stern warnings about the "misuse" of organs, as if they were designed strictly for reproduction. References abound in the critical literature to the 1985 *Discover* article which refers to the "fragile anus" and the "rugged vagina" (Treichler 1988b, 37)—only one of which, in an apparently unconscious reversal of gender stereotype, can stand up to the *really* rugged penis. It is vital to remember that AIDS was conceptualized as a "gay disease" *despite* the knowledge, in the first year of the epidemic, that "men and women, straights as well as gays," were affected (Perrow and Guillen 1990, 3).[6]

Homophobia has not only influenced the content of "expert" medical discourse but also structured its omissions, that is, whose problems were defined as "the" problem and whose were delayed, excluded, or constructed in relation to others' needs. The homophobic perception of AIDS as the "gay plague" harmed heterosexuals as well as gay men, lesbians, and bisexuals, fatally delaying research, education, and consciousness-raising. Women's needs were especially neglected. Data on women's treatment are still inadequate, since women are excluded from many clinical trials in order to avoid possible harm to potential fetuses (Faden, Kass, and McGraw 1996). This lack of information reflects the broader situation for women in general and lesbians in particular. The 1997 National Lesbian and Gay Health Association annual health conference "discussed the cycle in which lesbian research seems trapped" (Johnson 1997, 27). On the one hand, it is difficult to obtain funding for "lesbian-specific studies because no national data exists [sic] that demonstrates the need for such research" (27). Yet on the other hand, without that data "researchers cannot get the funding to undertake the kind of broad-based study that would show the diversity of the lesbian community and specific health needs" (27).

Whether one regards this general situation as an instance of deliberate sexism or not, it is important to realize that within the context of many other sexist practices in health care, it can only serve to perpetuate existing disadvantages to women. Women have been denied disability benefits because common manifestations of HIV specific to women have not been adequately documented in research, though many practitioners are well aware of them (ACT UP 1990, Byron 1991, Corea 1992). As a result, many women were affected by the lag in setting treatment standards for AIDS-related gynecological problems (Faden, Kass, and McGraw 1996).

Moreover, the medical concepts of HIV in women which finally did develop were subject to the influence of misogyny. Women were understood not as whole persons, or even as patients in our own right, but rather as "vectors of infection"—vaginas capable of infecting men sexually, or uteruses harboring the virus for transmission to innocent fetuses[7]—while being "accused of spreading a disease they were told they couldn't get" (Corea 1992, 176). In short, homophobic perceptions of AIDS, coupled with medical and social sexism, reinforced and exacerbated other sexist and homophobic beliefs and practices, while reinforcing the normative status of the heterosexual male in medicine as in the broader social world. On the surface, HIV may have seemed initially to enhance the illusory status of female heterosexuality as an identity certified by nature; however, it actually fueled and gave new forms to the mistrust and devaluation of women.

Even in the absence of overtly homophobic attitudes, the marginal status of lesbians, bisexuals, and gay men contributes to medical misconceptions regarding HIV and AIDS, owing to ignorance about gay lives and gay sexual practices. Researchers often conceptualize gay men as "a homogeneous population" (Patton 1985, 26), despite significant variations (both individual and group, for example, rural versus urban) in drug use, sexual behaviors, and other risk factors. Self-perceptions of sexual identity are strongly influenced by cultural background. Yet medical and broader social notions of sexual identity tend to assume sexual categories as perceived in white Euro-American middle-class culture. These assumptions, when brought to research efforts, result in inattention to or misunderstandings of specific sexual practices, which in turn lead to misconceived transmission risk information (Alonso and Koreck 1989). This cultural phenomenon is not readily addressed in medical science. Scientists and physicians are "presumed to be the 'authority' on which forms of sex might be 'safe'" (Patton 1985, 139), yet this authority is unwarranted, given the extent of medical ignorance regarding gay sexuality and identity.

And if medical science is ill informed about gay male sexual practices and their relation to HIV, it is even more so about the sexual practices of lesbians and bisexual women. Dr. Charles Schable of the Centers for Disease Control (CDC) made the now infamous assessment that there was no need "to study [HIV transmission among] lesbians because 'lesbians don't have much sex'" (Leonard 1990, 113)[8]—this in a statement to the lesbian magazine *Visibilities*. In the data that the CDC did compile, the only women classified as lesbians were those who had not had sex with a man since 1977 (Byron 1991, 28), yet in "an ongoing Kinsey study, 46 percent of the self-identified lesbians surveyed reported having sex with a man since 1980" (Leonard 1990, 114).

Moreover, when physicians do the reporting, it may be their own assumptions about a woman's sexual orientation which get recorded. Given the presumption of heterosexuality, Zoe Leonard reports, "it is very likely that most women . . . will never even be asked if they have had sex with other women. . . . [T]he CDC found it impossible to categorize nearly 700 out of 5,000 women because they couldn't determine their sexual behaviors from the report forms" (1990, 115). Furthermore, given the lack of research on HIV manifestations in women, some women who have not been diagnosed accurately will not be included in the statistics (Leonard 1990, 116). Thus, deep confusion at the most basic level—about which women are lesbians, and even which women have AIDS—has resulted in a severe dearth of information on HIV transmission and status among lesbians, and lesbians cannot necessarily trust what information there is.

Yet another statistical and conceptual problem is the CDC's use of hierarchically ranked categories of risk. For example, intravenous drug use outranks other possible modes of transmission, creating a potential for inaccurate results, as Leonard notes: "If you are a lesbian IVDU [intravenous drug user] with an IVDU partner, the possibility of woman-to-woman transmission would be ignored and you would be counted solely as an IVDU, even if you never shared needles" (115). Regardless of whether government agencies have deliberately neglected lesbians and bisexual women in the epidemic, the consequences are the same.

What should one make of these examples of oppressive practices, attitudes, and misconceptions in various aspects of medicine? Do they indicate profound problems in the institution of "medicine itself," or are they mere, though unfortunate, aberrations from "good" medicine? Are they "science as usual" or "bad science" (Harding 1986)? Is it not possible that providers' refusal to treat people with AIDS, their blame and fear of people with AIDS, and the failure to recognize chosen family members can be rectified with *better* medicine, more attention to good medical science, a little more objectivity in dealing with patients, and better medical education? That moralistic "medical" pronouncements are a misuse of medical language for rhetorical purposes and not a problem of medicine at all? That pathologizing gay identity and ignoring gay sexuality can be remedied simply by greater scientific accuracy, rehabilitating unavoidably unruly discourses and practices? In the next section I respond to these questions, giving an account of the privileged status of medical conceptualizations of difference and arguing that this privilege itself must be remedied, not merely the specific notions that exemplify it.

Medicine as Cultural Myth

Recent advances in drug treatments for HIV exposure and seropositivity have brought new problems in their wake. "Triple drug therapy," combining protease inhibitors with other anti-infectives, has been shown to reduce greatly the amount of virus in blood and lymph tissues; in some cases the virus eventually becomes almost undetectable (Brown 1997). Another treatment, "postexposure therapy," developed first for health care workers exposed to the virus through accidental needle sticks, has been shown to reduce transmission risks by 79 percent ("CDC Wrestles" 1997, "Corrections" 1997, Okie 1997). As a result, it has become more widely available and is sometimes requested after rape or unprotected consensual sex. David Barr, treatment education director of Gay Men's Health Crisis in New York, worries that "offering preventive drug treatment might relay 'mixed messages,' making people think they could engage in unsafe sex and worry about the consequences afterward" (Okie 1997, 15). His concern is not groundless: though more information is needed, one study of "men who have sex with men" found that "eighteen percent said that in engaging in unsafe sex, they believed that if they became infected, the new drug treatment would prevent them from becoming infected" (Keen 1997, 27).[9]

This dangerous faith in medicine is congruent with broader cultural assumptions about the status and value of medicine. Janice Raymond argues that "medicine functions as religion," and its vision of moral order "promotes anti-feminist beliefs, symbols, social memories, and churchly structures" (1982, 197). This patriarchal religion proclaims, "Outside the church there is no salvation" (209). Raymond's analysis can be used to explain the inferior or outsider status of holistic medicine, lay midwifery, feminist self-help groups, and some community AIDS research groups, all of which have been pronounced heretical by that church: not merely do these approaches violate institutional rules of knowledge and expertise, but they violate its vision of moral order as well.

This moral vision is not only anti-feminist, as Raymond suggests, but also deeply heterosexist; yet women or gay and bisexual men may wish to partake nonetheless because of its promise to restore order in a chaotic and sometimes terrifying world. Moreover, when medicine undermines one's sense of agency or integrity—which in the case of AIDS only compounds the enormous vulnerability of illness and loss—it is not surprising that a sense of helplessness might result. It is not pathology alone that has an existential dimension; so does the medical offer of help and healing, or even the perception that such help is possible where no such promise has been extended. This appeal may be very powerful to precisely those whose helplessness has been fostered by medical discourse.

One of the central tasks of religion is to provide myths that express a society's deepest values, those that structure its beliefs and practices. Medical discourse embodies (both literally and figuratively) a social mythology, and a crucial part of the story it tells involves the nature and meaning of social difference. It categorizes people into groups based on traits thought to be biologically based or physiologically manifested, such as gender, sexual orientation, race, age, and level of physical ability. Medical concepts of difference have an exalted status owing to the association of medicine with science, which is perceived as detached, objective, inherently unbiased. Yet not only do scientific "facts" regarding difference influence social practices, but they also are frequently based on an implicit norm whose reference points include heterosexual maleness, as exemplified by the "fragile anus/rugged vagina" doctrine.

Thus medical science and practice convey moral and political judgments which often serve the interests of the privileged, reassuring them of the rightness and inevitability of their social position, and doing so at the expense of those who already face social disadvantages—as when medical discourse is employed in arguments against gay civil rights legislation.[10] Political judgments using medical discourse can appear to be grounded in scientific objectivity, with its paramount epistemic authority, so that challenges to medical ideologies of difference may be seen as attempts by "special interest groups" to regulate science.[11] Objecting to the implicit homophobia of the "fragile anus/rugged vagina" concept is thus made to seem roughly analogous to claiming discrimination against diabetics because their doctors deny them donuts.

Recall Michel Foucault's historical overview of the developing ideological functions of medicine (1975). In valorizing scientific objectivity, the modern era fostered society's medicalization, with medicine replacing the church as the repository of social order. In this process, complex social forces, manifested in the health of individuals, were represented as discrete phenomena, the disconnected and seemingly random pathologies of individual organisms.

Foucault argues that what was important and new in the epistemology of the gaze was its status as a mode of truth both individual and specific yet objective and detached. This model separated knower and known, so that the object of study became the Other, and knowledge was radically detached from feeling, emotion, and experience. Seeking liberation from bias, the gaze metaphor effaces any active participation, involvement, or vested interest in the construction of knowledge, and casts the body, its experiences, and sensations as the passive and insensate Other.

The epistemic maneuver maximizing the distance between doctor and patient was not merely metaphorical but made literal when stethoscopes were invented to permit the doctor to hear a woman's heartbeat undisturbed by the sensation of her breasts against his face, thus expunging the unacknowledged and disturbing subjectivity of the doctor as well as the patient. With the advent of modern medicine, it is no longer sin or spiritual corruption that presents an obstacle to knowledge but physicality itself, the physicality of both doctor and patient, so that mediation is required. Foucault writes: "It is no longer shame that prevents contact . . . not the innocence, but the disgrace, of the body" (163)—a disgrace based on indeterminacy, its dark secrets requiring "instrumental mediation" to be known (164). Such mediation offers mastery in another sense beyond that of knowledge. Detachment not only promotes the discovery of hidden truths but also offers the physician insulation from the suffering, pain, and frailty which the patient represents.[12]

In this epistemic process, medicine acquires the status of cultural healer, a purity that is epistemically rather than religiously or spiritually certified, and that helps to resolve society's deep ambivalence toward science and technology, so frequently perceived as out of control. Based on this epistemic certification, medicine serves as the locus of ritual for creating, maintaining, and restoring social order. Health becomes a metaphor for self-control and merit (Crawford 1984), with particular applications, as I suggested earlier, for women of all sexual orientations, and gay and bisexual men.

Iris Young helps to clarify how this metaphoric value of health has profound implications for the relation between justice and health (1990). She argues that medical discourse and traditional accounts of justice share epistemic principles which perpetuate injustice. She is concerned with the persistence of oppression based on race, gender, sexual orientation, and other categories, despite the "discursive commitment to equality" that characterizes recent history (124). Oppressive attitudes still persist through "everyday habits and cultural meanings of which people are for the most part unaware" (124). She attributes these habits and attitudes to the largely unconscious "basic security system" of individuals, arguing that attitudes toward social groups function as part of one's sense of identity and "ontological integrity" (131).

Young distinguishes between "practical consciousness" or affect (which I understand to include the psychoanalytic concept of the individual unconscious, though conceptualized in relation to the broader social context) and "discursive consciousness" (which includes socially articulated values, goals, and intentions). The dread or loathing of difference or Otherness is a fear of "border ambiguity" (145), which Young argues is particularly significant in relation to homophobia. Sexual orientation can be perceived as the "most permeable" of social borders: race and gender are perceived as immutable physical characteristics, which cannot be changed through contact with members of other groups or through acts of will, though no such "specific characteristics" mark off sexual orientation (146). Thus anyone may become this Other, perhaps through the "corruption" of the Other's mere proximity. For Young, such anxieties suggest that increasing discursive clarity about sexual orientation will not in itself undermine homophobia: "[A]nyone at all can become gay, especially me, so the only way to defend my identity is to turn away with irrational disgust" (146).

The individually felt need to shore up ontological borders between Self and Other reflects broader cultural ideologies. Young situates medical science in the context of the historical association of "despised groups with the body, setting them outside the homogeneity of the nation" (111). Nineteenth-century categories of pathology presented socially constructed differences as truths of nature and classified them hierarchically. The result was "theories of human physical, moral, and aesthetic superiority, which presumed the young white bourgeois man as the norm" (130).

A crucial part of these theories were tenets about the nature of knowledge, its social value, and who had the capacity for it. Alison Jaggar defines normative dualism as "the belief that what is especially valuable about human beings is a particular 'mental' capacity, the capacity for rationality" (1983, 28). The social status of the medical profession lent support to this notion. Intelligence, conceived as the capacity for reasoning, was associated with the most privileged—white, heterosexual, middle- and upper-class males—in contrast to socially devalued groups, who were supposedly ruled by passion, emotion, or the body rather than the constraints of reason. "The unifying structure of that reason, which presumed a knowing subject purified of sensous immersion in things, made possible the objectification of other groups, and their placement under a normalizing gaze" (Young 1990, 130).

Young's indictment of the oppressive influences of medical authority is primarily historical. The AIDS epidemic, however, reveals that while medicine has the potential to help demystify homophobic notions and irrational fears and prejudice around AIDS, it also continues to support an oppressive social climate for lesbians, gay men, and bisexuals. This role in perpetuating oppression is not merely a matter of outmoded doctrines which eventually will be corrected through the progress of medical science. The problem is far deeper, owing to the socially sanctioned power of medicine to justify itself. The kinds of harms I have discussed, as well as broader social manifestations of homophobia, are rendered invisible by the cultural authority of medicine, or presented as inevitable, morally appropriate, or even the consequences "they" bring on themselves.

Sexual Oppression and Erotophobia

Thus far I have discussed tacit and overt medical norms regarding women and gay and bisexual men, who disproportionately experience certain health risks and health care needs, which then expose them to risks associated with health care itself, including its moral/political judgments. There is a further link: these groups are particularly subject to judgments on their sexual behaviors or "natures." I contend that sexual stereotyping is one of the hallmarks of oppression, by which I mean not merely the cultural association of a group with specific sexual tendencies or ways of being, but a widely recognized sexual image of that group which is connected to material and psychological harms inflicted on its members differentially.

That image may be a hypersexualized one, as in the case of African American men (hooks 1992) or gay and bisexual men (Mohr 1998, White 1996), subjecting them to criminal penalties for consensual sex (miscegenation and sodomy laws), and to hate crimes such as lynching and gay bashing (and possibly to higher conviction rates and harsher sentences for sex crimes such as rape). A group's image may be an entirely desexualized one, as it is for women with disabilities, who are even more vulnerable to rape and abuse than are nondisabled women (Krotoski, Nosek, and Turk 1996). Sexual images of women tend to be contradictory, imposing double binds such as the familiar prude/slut dichotomy which damns a woman if she does and damns her if she doesn't.[13] There is hardly an aspect of women's lives, from personal safety to relationships to the workplace to a woman's deepest feelings about herself, that is untouched by these images and the practices they support. Sexual images also take specific forms according to age, class, ethnicity, sexual orientation, and so on.

Whereas these sexual images and their political significance for particular groups have received a great deal of attention, their connection to one another and their status as a hallmark of oppression have not. As a result of the feminist work on sexual images of women and their relation to material practices, it is now possible—and, I would argue, strategically important—to begin an analysis that would connect women's sexual oppression to that of other groups, while attending carefully to the specifics of each group's experience.

A useful concept for such an analysis is erotophobia, as articulated by Cindy Patton (1985). Although it may in some contexts operate independently of social group differentiation, it is also an important dynamic in the notion of sexual oppression that I am suggesting. She defines erotophobia as:

the terrifying, irrational reaction to the erotic which makes individuals and society vulnerable to psychological and social control in cultures where pleasure is strictly categorized and regulated. Each component of sexuality—sexual practice, desire, and sexual identity—constitutes a particular type of relationship between the individual and society, providing gripping opportunities for different forms of erotophobic repression. (103)

Patton uses this concept primarily in a discussion of social policies and sexual politics, but she also extends it to the politics of medical knowledge. I understand erotophobia (like homophobia) to consist not only of explicit declarations of pathology, but also of other practices and attitudes which more subtly reflect cultural taboos against sexual practices, desires, and identities.

Patton's analysis can be situated within the approach she terms "the sexual unorthodoxy," as well as the emerging field of queer theory.[14] I apply her concept to its manifestations in each of the four aspects of medicine I identified earlier, in order to show that bioethics should incorporate analysis of the cultural politics of sexuality, that feminist and anti-oppression analysis more broadly can benefit from the insights of queer theory, and that queer theory must continue to employ feminist analysis.

In the first aspect of medicine, health care providers may manifest erotophobia in their unwillingness or inability to provide information or interview patients about sexuality and related health concerns, and in giving patients incomplete or inaccurate information. In 1996 the *Journal of the American Medical Association* reported on research indicating that "only 11% to 37% of primary care physicians routinely take a sexual history from their new adult patients" (Keen 1996, 19). As a result, "doctors often fail to screen, diagnose, or treat important medical problems," particularly in gay and lesbian patients (19). Other studies indicate that only 44 percent of gay men and 33 percent of lesbians disclose their sexual identity to doctors (19). A cultural context of erotophobia influences both doctors and patients, undermining care, when doctors fail to address sexual issues clearly, and patients are unable to speak openly about sexual experiences and concerns. And to the extent that heterosexism or sexist attitudes toward female sexualities influence doctors' assumptions about and treatment of patients, again, erotophobia undermines decent care. In general, medical erotophobia reinforces wider social stigmas.

Once again, however, this problem may be dismissed, at least as a flaw of the institution of medicine itself, if it consists mainly of unfortunate attitudes and practices on the part of some individuals. Earlier I noted various examples of physicians' mistreatment of people with AIDS. Patton shows why these examples must not be dismissed as isolated incidents: erotophobia is a cultural norm that prescribes certain social relationships while proscribing others, rather than an idiosyncrasy or a neurosis which happens to afflict some individuals—which can be seen in manifestations of erotophobia in the next aspect of medicine.

Basic access to information about sexuality, particularly for adolescents, is a critical issue in the popular representation of medical information, the second aspect of medicine. Frances Kunreuther, director of a New York social service agency for gay youths, notes, "The problems with educating teens about AIDS is complicated by the difficulty that adults have in speaking to adolescents about sex, especially homosexuality" (Wolinsky 1991). More generally, there is a widespread social reluctance to publicize information regarding specific sexual practices, contraception, and HIV risk reduction for fear of "condoning" or "promoting" homosexuality, "promiscuity," or premarital or extramarital sex.

This fear leads to efforts to instill other fears in young people. "Abstinence-only" sex education curricula are being implemented throughout the United States as a result of the 1996 Welfare Reform Law's provision of $250 million in grants for such programs (Saliba 1997, 2). *No Second Chance,* a video used in "Sex Respect," one of the most popular of these programs, offers the following dialogue:

> Student [to nurse-inspector]: What if I want to have sex before I get married?
> Instructor: Well, I guess you'll just have to be prepared to die. And you'll probably take with you your spouse and one or more of your children. (Saliba 1997, 2)

"Sex Respect" also warns, "No one can deny that nature is making . . . a comment on sexual behavior through the AIDS and herpes epidemics"

(Saliba 1997, 2). Along with these punitive ideas at the core of abstinence-only programs are others which are inaccurate and reactionary: "One program . . . tells students that HIV can 'pass through the pores of a latex condom.' . . . Some of the programs also portray minority teens as promiscuous and needy" ("Sex Education" 1997, 18). Perhaps the most damaging aspect of the programs, however, is their prohibition of information about safer sex and contraception—despite many studies confirming not only that both condoms and safer sex information are effective in preventing HIV transmission (Okie 1997, A8), but also that comprehensive sex education does not increase sexual activity (Saliba 1997, 2).

For adults as well as teenagers, the difficulties in access to information may be compounded by strong societal incentives to deny same-sex practices or identity. In Sarah Schulman's novel *People in Trouble* (1990), Jeffrey, an AIDS hotline volunteer, speaks with a man who identifies himself as heterosexual and claims generally to have practiced safer sex, yet seems very worried about AIDS. As Jeffrey tells a friend later, despite his reassurances to the caller,

> the guy wouldn't get off the phone. He kept hemming and hawing saying, "Are you sure? Are you sure?" So I finally got the message and gave him what he wanted. "Are you having sex with men?" I asked. "No, no, no not me," he says. "Are you sure?" I say. "Are you sure you didn't do it just once? Just to see what it was like . . . because you were really horny . . . [and] you didn't realize what you were doing and before you realized it, some faggot . . ." "You know," he says. "Something is coming back to me now that you mention it. Yeah, I think I was really plastered. Totally smashed." Like that. . . .
>
> You have to give them every excuse in the world so they can tell you what they did without admitting to being gay. (75)

As this fictional episode illustrates, there is pressure to deny same-sex practice or identity not merely to others but to oneself as well. The caller here seems to have internalized homophobic and erotophobic attitudes; he struggles with acknowledging his sexual practices not just to the faceless hotline volunteer but even to himself. With much prodding from Jeffrey, he does manage eventually to get at least basic information. Without such help in the real world, many people do not overcome these difficulties.

A striking example of erotophobic taboo was the controversy over then–Surgeon General Joycelyn Elders's comments about masturbation in a discussion period following her 1994 World AIDS Day speech at the United Nations. Rob Clark, of the Society for the Psychological Study of Social Issues, addressed the following remarks to Elders: "It seems to me the campaign against AIDS has already destroyed many taboos about discussion of sex in public. It seems to me that there still remains a taboo against the discussion about masturbation. . . . [W]hat do you think are the prospects of a more explicit discussion and promotion of masturbation?" Elders replied:

I think you already know that I'm a very strong advocate of a comprehensive health education program if you will, starting at a very early age. I feel that it should be age appropriate, it should be complete, and we need to teach our children the things that they need to know. And we know that many of our parents have difficulty teaching certain things. And for that reason, to make sure all of our children are informed, I've always felt that we should make it a part of our school. . . .

As per your specific question in regard to masturbation, I think that is something that is a part of human sexuality and it's a part of something that perhaps should be taught. But we've not even taught our children the very basics. And I feel that we have tried ignorance for a very long time, and it's time we try education. ("Comments" 1994)

Elders's statement may have been vague, but it was certainly benign, and indeed even sensible. She was forced to resign for many controversial comments (not all of which were about sexuality) made during her tenure as surgeon general; this incident was generally regarded as the proverbial last straw. Nonetheless, her dismissal by President Clinton and the ensuing media commentary reflect precisely those erotophobic taboos which she and others criticized on World AIDS Day, ironically underscoring their point. Afterwards, some commentators responded with moral outrage, while those who were more liberal treated her as an object of ridicule; few attempted to defend her. This response reveals cultural priorities apparent in the epidemic: it is better to avoid mentioning the taboo sexual practice of masturbation, despite its status as the *only* altogether "safe" sexual practice, than to seem to condone a forbidden, "degenerate" sexual practice.[15]

Moreover, what may appear on the surface as cultural embarrassment about sexual matters, or generalized sexual "prudishness," actually reflects deeper values at the intersection of erotophobia, homophobia, and sexism. Whatever the lasting effects of the "sexual revolution" really were, they did not include a generalized tolerance of or openness to the range of human sexual practices, not even among young people. For example, a psychiatrist in Bethesda, Maryland, "is often told by young boys who have fathered babies that [masturbation] 'is gay; you can't be gay so you got to dip your wick [have vaginal intercourse] to get off'" (Welsh 1994). Sex educators note seemingly convoluted notions of sexual morality: to some religious young people, anal intercourse does not count as sex "because it is not losing your virginity," and masturbation is "a far greater sin than intercourse" (Welsh 1994). Yet these attitudes are not difficult to explain. While the parents and religious leaders of these young people surely would not condone their view of anal intercourse, it does indicate how the symbolic aspects of sexuality frequently take precedence over the practical consequences. In short, the masturbation taboo reflected in the response to Elders reveals the normative status of heterosexual masculinity, the generalized suspicion of erotic pleasure, and the particularly sexist and homophobic neglect of sexually active young gay and bisexual men and heterosexual women, who face a higher risk of transmission through either vaginal or anal intercourse than do heterosexual males.

Erotophobia, then, restricts the transmission of AIDS information, undermines people's ability to seek or to absorb such information, and distorts information in the mass media, such as the conflation of sexual identity with high-risk practices, discussed earlier. It is also apparent in the conflation of medical and moral "pathology" discussed earlier. But what of the third aspect of medicine—medical conceptualizations themselves? In what sense could erotophobia be said to be influential here?

"The cultural erotophobia which conflates practice, desire, and identity" (Patton 1985, 135) suggests not just that sexual identities are immutable but that sexual practices are not subject to change either; thus risk reduction is perceived as impossible, especially for gay men. This perception not only interferes with the accuracy and effectiveness of AIDS information; it also has influenced the ways in which "the facts" of the epidemic have been understood. Thus some misconceptions and omissions, such as the lack of information about lesbians and HIV, stem from cultural erotophobia, even in the absence of overtly oppressive beliefs or intent. Despite the fact that scientific discourses on sexuality have proliferated as never before, producing a vast array of information, it could still be said that erotophobia may exert subtle influence on which problems, and whose problems, get attention in research; on which groups are seen as mainstream, their needs central, and whose needs and concerns are seen as marginal or exceptional.

Patton cites a "hierarchy of sexual deviance" as an "axiom" of erotophobia (1985, 133). This hierarchy helps to explain some of the omissions and distortions in HIV discourse which I have noted. Not only does it help to account for the seemingly convoluted notions of sexual morality held by some adolescents, but also it suggests that what appear to be medical judgments are actually moral judgments about sexual behavior—which at a still deeper level are another way to pathologize social difference. Beneath the stated concern for the medical ramifications of sexual behavior are moral judgments that certify the medical, hence moral, correctness of white, middle-class, monogamous, married heterosexuality, and prescribe a whole set of gender relations in marriages.

Erotophobia, then, connects directly to the fourth aspect of medicine through the myth of selflessness, discussed in the previous chapter: the erasure of selves and the delegitimation of subjectivities through the pathologizing of certain identities and groups; and the explicit behavioral and sexual norms that legitimate female sexuality only as it conforms to status quo gender relations, and more broadly prescribe unselfishness, existing for the sake of others, as a veritable gynecological virtue. The medical construction of women as mothers consigns female sexualities to the realm of sexual deviance as well, unless redeemed by childbearing, thus suggesting that lesbians are particularly deviant among women.

Sexual deviance, then, is not merely a statistical concept. It is a moral concept based on conservative notions of the family,[16] encoding misogynist and homophobic fears of the "contaminating" presence of lesbians, bisexuals, gay men, and heterosexual women outside the institution of marriage. It also expresses and enforces patriarchal and heterosexist expectations of the behaviors of these groups. The institution of medicine contributes substantially to this moral/political norm's expression and enforcement, and medicine's scientific grounding offers a justification far more effective than the nonscientific justifications which were formerly sufficient.

Medicine, then, is not simply science applied to the goal of healing, but a powerful form of moral and political authority which contributes significantly to oppression, despite the benefits it has also brought to members of oppressed groups. Yet movements based on the identities of these groups clearly establish greater access to health care among their top political priorities: for basic physical survival, as well as improved physical health, functioning, and quality of life; and because of specific health risks and needs associated with these groups. The next two chapters explore that topic.

ॐ

3

Real Selves: Illness and Other Ontological Assaults

There may be no single factor that influences our health more than the circumstances of our birth. Many readers may be inclined to think first of genetics here. Individuals, however, are born not only with distinct genetic mixes which connect them to their families, but also into circumstances, including social group categories, which strongly affect both health status and access to care. Oppression manifests itself in, among other ways, poorer prospects for health, safety, and bodily integrity for some social groups relative to others. This problem has three elements which together constitute a powerful social interference with the health and well-being of many members of society.

First, members of oppressed groups may have a greater need for health care than others. For example, African Americans face differentials in life expectancy, infant and general mortality rates, vulnerability to assault and murder, and rates of disability, AIDS, hypertension, tuberculosis, cancer, and other diseases.[1] A large body of literature attributes these and other health differentials to social problems including racism, violence, poverty, classism, sexism, stress, unresolved grief from premature losses experienced in urban African American communities, militarization of the economy, and disabled women's particular vulnerability to abuse.[2]

Second, a variety of barriers undermine oppressed groups' access to care. Some of these include gender and racial disparities in access to health insurance (Nechas and Foley 1994, Nelson and Nelson 1996); hospital closings in poor black communities and cutbacks in Medicaid funding (A. Davis 1990); and black women's difficulties in obtaining drug treatment, care from private providers, and prenatal care when HIV positive (Battle 1990, Killion 1990, Richie 1990). Contributors to Annette Dula and Sara Goering's *"It Just Ain't Fair": The Ethics of Health Care for African-Americans* (1994) focus on African Americans who are poor, homeless, or HIV positive, or who are grandparents caring for grandchildren who have lost parents to AIDS. Together they present a compelling argument that many social factors interact to present multiple obstacles to health care.

Third, as Chapters 1 and 2 have shown in the context of obstetrics, gynecology, violence against women, and HIV, access to care itself can be a mixed blessing. For example, Medicaid, the main source of health care funding for poor patients, is frequently criticized for substandard and fragmented care (Beardsley 1990, Nechas and Foley 1994). Sue Fisher confirms differential treatment of female patients based on socioeconomic class (1986). Care available for the poor at large urban hospitals can be dehumanizing, with practitioners expressing cynical or judgmental attitudes (Killion 1990, Ferguson 1994).

Furthermore, care for oppressed groups is often based on insufficent research, owing to the status of the middle-class, able-bodied white male as normative research subject. There is often a gap in funding for research on diseases such as sickle-cell anemia which tend not to affect the "normative" group (Mechanic 1984). Efforts to protect women from potential reproductive hazards associated with research function to exclude women from clinical studies (Merton 1996, Nechas and Foley 1994). Some research addresses health concerns common to both genders, such as substance abuse and heart disease, but fails to address different manifestations or treatment implications for women (Nechas and Foley 1994). Medical education also tends to focus on the male, treating women's health issues as secondary (Nechas and Foley 1994).

People with disabilities experience multiple problems with care. Medicine tends to desexualize those with disabilities, especially women, leaving patients at a loss for much-needed treatment, information, and support, especially on issues such as contraception, sexually transmitted diseases, and menopause (Nosek 1996a, Welner 1996, O'Toole 1996). This general problem is compounded for lesbians with disabilities (O'Toole 1996).

Women with disabilities face a greater risk of abuse than other women, yet one study reports that providers may discount the reports of women with disabilities, or fail to recognize signs of abuse (Nosek 1996a). Furthermore, care for women with disabilities is often heavily laced with paternalism (Gill 1996, Rogers 1996, Wendell 1996). All of these examples present a disturbing picture of the risks for oppressed groups of medical stigmatization, control, and mistreatment or inadequate treatment, reinforcing the stigma and constraints that oppression perpetuates in other aspects of life.

Activists on various fronts continue to struggle for broader access to health care for those suffering from HIV, urban violence, unwanted pregnancy (teenage and otherwise), abortion clinic violence and other problems of access to abortion, and a host of poverty-related health problems, including maternal and infant mortality and morbidity. The philosophical literature also reflects this concern. Here, access to health care is usually identified as the central issue in the relation of justice to health, and many philosophers offer rationales for increased access. Yet if social group status influences need, complicates access, and links care to stigma and control, then the oppressive aspects of medicine, and the social interferences with both health and access, must be evaluated along with the benefits of medicine, both actual and potential.

Distribution is the dominant paradigm of justice in twentieth-century American analytic philosophy. Tom Beauchamp and James Childress's *Principles of Biomedical Ethics* (1979) identified justice as one of four central principles of bioethics. Taking their lead, bioethicists since then have tended to emphasize distributive justice over other aspects, applying the principle most often to issues of allocation.[3] This approach allows identification of the straightforwardly economic aspects of access, but offers no clear way to conceptualize more subtle barriers to care, the multitude of social influences that give rise to the health care needs of members of oppressed groups, or problems with their care, especially those that go beyond the doctor-patient relationship. This paradigm fails to capture the social relations of medicine, including the moral authority that enables it to stigmatize the very social groups that are already marginalized. Its neglect of such important aspects of power is a serious weakness of the larger paradigm, a failing that, moreover, manifests itself in both conservative and liberal theories of justice in health and health care.

Iris Young calls for a reconceptualization of justice recognizing that social group difference structures our lives in many ways, creating enormous disparities in power, influence, and overall well-being; that oppression is a key aspect of injustice; and that justice therefore requires structural changes to society (1990). Such an approach would permit long-overdue moral reflection on neglected topics in health and justice. I offer a concept of selfhood as an avenue into this broader understanding of justice. I have argued that common operations of medical discourse are destructive to the selfhood of women as well as gay and bisexual men. In this chapter I extend that argument to the operations of liberal philosophical discourse, particularly as it influences bioethics, and work toward a reconceptualized health-justice relation by contrast, through a detailed critique of three liberal theorists. Both the critical and the positive strands of the argument are needed, on the one hand, to trace the inegalitarian continuities between the discourses of medicine and bioethics, including certain epistemic principles, and on the other hand, to begin developing an alternative to the standard method. I use the material-semiotic approach to health developed in previous chapters, and advocate a material-semiotic model of the self as a corrective to the abstract, rationalist concept of personhood which dominates liberal theory. This model can provide a richer understanding of health issues as they are experienced by individuals in specific cultural contexts, counteracting medical devaluation of oppressed groups.

The kind of health care analysis that I propose has interesting ramifications for social and political philosophy more broadly. Rectifying inequities and meeting the needs of the disempowered in relation to health is quite likely to carry over into other areas as well, challenging the standard philosophical discussion of justice in health as a distributive problem, involving a clear tradeoff between health and other goods. This analysis also unsettles the standard liberal distinction between the natural and the social. It suggests that there is an important role for subjective experience and situated reflection in social policy, and that these modes of theorizing are valuable—necessary, even—for bioethics. My aim in this chapter, then, is to illustrate an approach that takes oppression as a central concern, emphasizing feminist and sexually inclusive standpoints in particular, and demonstrating the advantages of this method over standard liberal theories of access to health care.

This exploration also speaks to current questions in cultural studies work.

Because of the location of bioethics at the intersection of science and the humanities, its dual academic constituency, and its clear-cut immediacy, even urgency, for clients and activists, it offers a key opportunity for social dialogue and critique. At this site cultural analysis offers tools for articulating and advocating humanistic concerns (Poirier and Brauner 1988), for assisting the moral reflection of those in the medical field, and for challenging the political authority of science. For a cultural studies audience, this site, where immediate policy issues are being deliberated, presents a clear opportunity to bypass the tendency to theorize "the body" while neglecting the suffering of particular bodies (Wendell 1996, 44).

It will be useful here to survey liberal notions of human nature and selfhood, and epistemic continuities between liberalism and medicine, in order to clarify my departures from these views. Rationality, individualism, and self-interest are key elements in liberal views of human nature. Human essence is defined (both descriptively and normatively) as the capacity for rationality, the shared trait that is understood to ground moral dignity (Benhabib 1986, 411). Alison Jaggar points out that rationality "is conceived as a property of individuals rather than groups," a "metaphysical assumption [that] is sometimes called abstract individualism because it conceives of human individuals in abstraction from any social circumstances" (1983, 28–29). Furthermore, "rationality . . . is assumed to be a capacity that is possessed in approximately equal measure at least by all men" (29), and rationality is, in one way or another, linked with individuals' self-interest, either as a basic motive shared by all or as the justification for the social contract (28–29). This abstract and rationalist view of the self can both obscure and reinforce the social privilege of some groups at the expense of others.

But on the material-semiotic view of the self which I advocate, subjective experience and emotion are part of human agency, along with reason. Personhood in general, and individuality in particular, are conditioned by physicality; human biology provides us with a range of limits and capacities affecting our daily choices, yet biology constantly interacts with social practice, so that the two exist in a dynamic relationship. This model recognizes that health states fluctuate over the course of a lifetime (in contrast to liberal theories which tend to assume a basic level of minimum health, treating serious illness, injury, or disability as aberrations or as erosions of

selfhood), and they vary greatly between individuals while reflecting individual circumstances and social factors within particular communities.
Thus, disability and serious health problems should be considered as part of
the human condition rather than as sources of special needs for only some
individuals (Wendell 1996). To put these characteristics of human existence
into the background of theory is to understand them from the serious limitations of a privileged perspective.[4] Not just individual health but any departure from it is socially constituted, and interacts with (other) socially
constituted erosions of autonomy and integrity. Like other aspects of selfhood, health is always and only constituted in relation to particular social
contexts. Moreover, this view departs from the individualism of liberal theory, asserting the centrality of connections with others to personhood.[5]

Iris Young argues that medical discourse and traditional accounts of
justice share epistemic principles that help to perpetuate injustice (1990).
Mainstream moral and political theory, as well as popular discourses of social justice, generally share medicine's epistemology of detachment, with
its conception of objectivity as distance and neutrality. There is a sense that
unbiased public policy, for example, requires giving all groups or individuals equal standing and weighing their interests accordingly. Differential
treatment of any kind is felt to be "preferential treatment," which is understood as unfair, inherently wrong. Yet the problem remains that different social groups may have different needs, and individuals may experience
certain harms differentially as members of a particular group; if so, differential treatment may be required to redress these harms.

"The scale of the gaze," Foucault's phrase for the epistemic standard of
medicine (1975), could equally describe the discourse of social justice. The
"view from nowhere" (Nagel 1986) symbolizes a detached, hence objective, model of knowledge, precisely because it avoids the perceptual limitations of any single perceiver at any single location. Yet this visual metaphor seems strikingly inappropriate, given that vision is inherently situated
in the specific and limited vantage point of a particular perspective (Bordo
1990).

Both medical discourse and the mainstream discourse of social justice
have denied any epistemic role to experience and feeling, both sensory and
emotive (Jaggar 1989), and to the individual and social circumstances that
mediate them. For example, attending to lesbians', bisexuals', and gay men's
experiences with medical discourse (which I do not separate from medi-

cal practice) fosters a profound conviction of the injustice of homophobia. Yet the "view from nowhere," which prescribes nonpreferential treatment for all, seems inadequate to dismantle the categories of social hierarchy imposed by the medical gaze—a task that is necessary to determine what justice requires of society in relation not only to health but also to the broader social status of oppressed groups, issues that activist movements have rightly claimed are connected.

Moreover, like the ideology of medicine, the mainstream conceptualization of justice upholds the Enlightenment valorization of reason not only as the utmost human value but as the essence of agency itself, the chief resource for the pursuit of human needs. From this perspective, it is reason and argumentation that bring about social change and liberation. Yet, as Iris Young points out, oppression persists despite a "discursive commitment to equality" in recent history (1990, 124). She argues that the distributive paradigm fails to conceptualize the significance of cultural imperialism, the overt and subtle devaluation of oppressed groups via cultural mythology. I suggest that it is not only the distributive focus of the mainstream concept of justice which obscures this phenomenon but also its rationalism, emphasizing reason and objectivity—or at least one version of it—to the detriment of other human capacities.[6] The notion of objectivity construed as detachment may help to establish the impermissibility of overt discrimination, but it does nothing to foster the knowledge of others' experience or the suspension of trust in the universality of one own's experience—attitudes that may be particularly difficult to achieve for members of privileged groups, who tend to minimize the significance of social group status, universalizing their experience or taking it as the norm from which Others depart.[7]

Maria Lugones writes of the ethnocentric (and by analogy sexist and homophobic, or perhaps heterocentric) tendency to universalize on the basis of one's own particular experience, if not owned as such:

> You do not see me because you do not see yourself and you do not see yourself because you declare yourself outside of culture. But declaring yourself outside of culture is self-deceiving. The deception hides your seeing only through the eyes of your culture. So dis-engagement is a radical form of passivity toward the ideology of the ethnocentric racial state which privileges the dominant culture as the only culture to "see

with" and conceives this seeing as to be done non–self-consciously. (1990, 51)

Such operations of ethnocentric racism are a form of cultural imperialism. For Lugones, moral and political questions are always also epistemic questions. Considered in the context of Foucault's metaphor, her argument also suggests that the central problem with "the scale of the gaze" is that the apparent freedom of the gaze to master all it surveys disguises its inherent confinement to surfaces, the expulsion not just of subjectivity from the realm of knowledge but of the seer's awareness of her own locatedness and acknowledgment of her particular social location. Privilege means not only not having to acknowledge the contents of one's perspective, but also not having to acknowledge that one inevitably has a perspective. I suggest that situated modes of analysis have much to offer bioethics; access, for example, must be understood from the viewpoints of members of oppressed groups, taking subjective perceptions into account, and the bias of privileged ways of perceiving the social world must not go unchallenged.

Before I begin my analysis of liberal theory in bioethics, it will be useful to distinguish "liberalism" in the political sense from the broader philosophical framework that encompasses the range of mainstream politics. David Gauthier and Norman Daniels exemplify the fairly broad political range among those currently working within the conceptual framework of liberalism which has dominated philosophy for centuries, with its familiar values such as liberty, equality, and individual rights. (I use the unqualified term "liberalism" to refer to the broad philosophical framework.)

The work of these theorists provides a special opportunity to reflect on access to health care within broader social visions, theories of justice or of morality and the legitimate constraints on self-interest: Daniels's work is congruent with, and perhaps even inspired by, John Rawls's *A Theory of Justice* (1971), while Gauthier's work on health care follows his own *Morals by Agreement* (1986).

Their work contrasts sharply on political grounds, offering an opportunity to examine theoretical continuities across political difference. There are two main contenders for the principle governing the distribution of health care (with variations in how each is formulated and the restrictions and special cases for each): market access to health care (that is, access determined by individual ability to pay), as in the United States, or some more egalitarian distribution, as in Great Britain or Canada. Gauthier falls into the former camp: his "Unequal Need" (1983) appeared in a Reagan administration commission report on access to health care, and his work reflects that conservative political climate. Daniels calls for a more egalitarian approach. He began *Just Health Care* in 1978, sharing a "public perception . . . that justice required improved access to health care" (1985, x).

Despite these political differences, however, their work may be criticized on similar grounds from the perspectives of activist health movements: for inappropriately attributing natural origins to particular goods, and for assuming a simplistic and inaccurate dichotomy between the natural and the social, which prevents the full recognition and moral evaluation of the influence of social practices on individual health. An especially problematic effect of this dichotomy is to obscure the social origin of practices that differentially harm members of oppressed groups, while making these harms appear to be "facts of nature." They also can be criticized for the different ways in which they take the existing health care system for granted in their theories of access.

A third work, that of Robert Dickman (1983), offers a critical assessment of one aspect of the existing system, focusing on the subjective aspects of health care for low-income patients, including its effects on self-esteem. Dickman assesses the political significance of this concern, extending the question of justice in health beyond the norm for liberal treatments. Yet without explicit attention to social group difference and its current and ongoing manifestations, even this work has serious limitations in addressing patients' lived experience of health care.

Gauthier's Contractarian Analysis

Gauthier's health care theory must first be situated in the context of his earlier work, which restricts the domain not only of justice but also of morality in general to rational individuals capable of benefiting others through past, present, or future contributions to the economy. I argue that this starting point builds in an "ableist" bias, which manifests itself quite clearly in Gauthier's health care theory, and is connected to a distinction between the natural and social so firmly drawn as to underestimate grossly the social causes of health problems.

In *Morals by Agreement,* Gauthier "defend[s] the traditional conception of morality as a rational constraint on the pursuit of individual interest" (1986, 2). Arguing that morality cannot be reduced to self-interest, he identifies impartiality as the key for justifying constraints on individuals' pursuit of their own interest. He endorses Rawls's view of society as "a cooperative venture for mutual advantage" (10).

Gauthier's version of the social contract includes only those who are more or less equal: "Only beings whose physical and mental capacities are either roughly equal or mutually complementary can expect to find cooperation beneficial to all. . . . Among unequals, one party may benefit most by coercing the other, and on our theory would have no reason to refrain. We may condemn all coercive relationships, but only within the context of mutual benefit can our condemnation appeal to a rationally grounded morality" (17). Restricting the social contract to those who are "rough equals" clearly excludes some parties. Gauthier does not find this framework overly restrictive, however, since he identifies "the rationality of the participants" (17) as sufficient basis for this equality, and sees Western society as having largely achieved some semblance of "a co-operative venture for mutual advantage" (17), a claim that becomes far less plausible when assessed from the standpoints of people of color or other members of oppressed groups.

For Gauthier, one clear meaning of mutual benefit is mutual contribution to the economy, an idea with serious ramifications for dealing with disability. Gauthier notes that medical technology has increased the number of people who receive benefits from others without "increasing the average level of well-being" (18), and who are thus outside the domain of morality as he understands it: "Such persons are not party to the moral relationships grounded by a contractarian theory" (18). He specifies that those he has in mind are not the elderly, who "have paid for their benefits by earlier productive activity," but rather disabled people who need "life-extending therapies" (18). In a footnote Gauthier writes, "Speaking euphemistically of enabling them [the non-elderly disabled] to live productive lives, when the services required exceed any possible products, conceals an issue which, understandably, no one wants to face" (18).

In "Unequal Need" (1983), Gauthier argues that justice does not require that society subsidize the cost of health care, except for those with substandard resources. The central tenets of his argument are as follows: Fair access is not necessarily equal access, and a just distribution of health care must be cost-effective; ordinary market provision of health care meets these requirements;[8] and tradeoffs between health care and other goods require clear limits on health care entitlements. In his view (he was writing in 1983), the actual distribution of resources in the United States is generally fair; "general social poverty" is not the case; and this society generally contributes to the good lives of its members—a view most persuasive, perhaps, to those who are privileged, but less than plausible when assessed in terms of social group differentials.

The metaphysical underpinnings of this argument bear close scrutiny. Gauthier identifies health as one of the primary goods, which John Rawls defines "as those 'things that every rational man is presumed to want. These goods normally have a use whatever a person's rational plan of life'" (Gauthier 1983, 180). This scheme, according to Gauthier, is an "individualistic and pluralistic characterization of the good," recognizing that there will be differences in life plans (180–81). The distribution of primary goods is clearly a significant aspect of justice, since they are necessary for individuals' pursuit of the good life. Quoting from Rawls, Gauthier categorizes primary goods as originating either "naturally" or "socially":

> "Rights and liberties, powers and opportunities, income and wealth" constitute the principal social primary goods; "health and vigor, intelligence and imagination" are natural goods. Underlying this distinction is the fact that the distribution of goods in the first group is essentially influenced, if not fully determined, by the particular features of a social system, and so may be brought under deliberate social control; however, distribution of goods in the second group is relatively immune to social control, at least of a planned kind. (181)

This distinction seems to be based on the understanding that as a member of a particular society, I have access to certain goods, some of which might be lost to me and others gained were I to move to another society whose policies and resources were different, while other kinds of goods seem less susceptible to such change.

Gauthier identifies health as a natural primary good "in significant respects" (182), though it has more in common with social primary goods than other natural primary goods do. It is "naturally based" (185), yet, "like a state of wealth, is largely socially conditioned and is alterable by deliberate, planned social intervention" (185). It is difficult to understand health as a unique kind of natural good. Perhaps Gauthier considers it, while alterable to some extent by social conditions, as linked to individual genetic fate in a way in which social goods are not (leaving aside the question of why genetic structure should be seen as completely "natural" in origin). Because health is susceptible to social intervention, however, Gauthier suggests that we are to consider it as if it were a social primary good; thus "the good society will enhance the health of its members to the greatest possible extent" (186)—at least insofar as maximizing health does not interfere unduly with efficiency or with the mutually beneficial character of society. Health is of *instrumental* value in pursuing the good life, which for Gauthier is to some extent defined relative to one's starting point in life, since the good life involves actualizing natural talents and capacities (185).

Gauthier's view of the nature of health as a good is based on his underlying conception of personhood. He distinguishes "between the status of an individual's condition of health and his or her abilities, interests, and traits of character. The latter we take to be constitutive of a particular individual" (184). Identity is constituted by relatively permanent components of character or personality: "We speak only partially metaphorically when we say of someone who undergoes marked alterations in character . . . that he or she is a different person. Such natural goods as intelligence, imagination, and industry, as constitutive features of a person's character, thus enter directly into individuality, making him or her that particular person" (184).

Thus it could be said that in Gauthier's view, abilities and interests are ontological/essential properties of the individual, while her state of (ill) health is not "similarly constitutive of individuality. A person who is handicapped or impaired is thought of as something less than his or her *real self*—less than the self who would emerge were the handicap or impairment overcome. Disease . . . is something that befalls a person, an accident in relation to nature or identity" (184). It is important to see that this notion of the "real self" is not merely descriptive but carries within it an implicit norm of health and able-bodiedness. This separation of health condition from identity seems plausible insofar as it captures the sense of the disabled person's claim, "I am not my disability."[9] It also captures the liberal intuition that identity has more to do with rationality, or the choices made by individuals, than with the nature of their circumstances.

Finally, Gauthier suggests that "what is essential to a particular person" is distinct "from what accidentally befalls a person": that is, "the way in which we distinguish what is essential . . . is affected by our beliefs about what is changeable through deliberate intervention" (184). This distinction "reflects a particular stage in the development of human technology" (184). He notes, for example, that as treatments have developed for leprosy, epilepsy, and consumption, these have come to be seen as "temporary, accidental diseases" rather than "permanent, constitutive conditions"; as a result, the people who have these conditions have been viewed differently as well.

Two aspects in particular of this concept of identity must be critically addressed: the distinction between natural and social goods, and the criteria for the features constitutive of selfhood. Both of these rest on problematic assumptions about the natural-social boundary.

It is not clear that the common distinction between natural and social goods used by Gauthier and others is altogether tenable. Gauthier considers intelligence and imaginative capacity ontological properties owing to their origin, their (relative) permanence, and their unquestioned status as natural objects. Each aspect of this view contains undefended and problematic assumptions.

First of all, Gauthier's reasoning obscures the impact of social policies and practices on individual characteristics. There may be biological aspects of "natural" goods such as intelligence and other capacities, yet these traits are nevertheless significantly influenced by prenatal access to goods that are clearly social in origin, including nutrition, adequate health care, and other basic life resources. Access to these goods is thus significantly influenced by social policies.

Although liberal theorists generally recognize that one's environment affects one's share of natural goods (in terms of both origin and perpetuation or enhancement), this effect seems to be understood as fairly minimal in scope. This is not an uncommon view in our society. Some students are labeled less intelligent than others (on the basis of standardized tests, for example), and variations in test scores or in educational achievement measured on the basis of grades are often attributed to individual short-comings or failures—differences in "native" intelligence, or weakness of character made manifest by lack of effort. Yet the dramatic inequities in resource allocations among various groups in society can be seen as a strong influence on these "individual traits." Jonathan Kozol reports, for example, an average student-counselor ratio of 150 to 1 in suburban Chicago schools versus 400 to 1 in Chicago; sixty thousand volumes in an average suburban library versus thirteen thousand in the city; and $90,000 more in funding per class at some suburban Chicago schools than in their urban counter-parts.[10] Such inequities are likely to result in the very disparities in intelligence ratings which are thought to be "natural," outside human control.

A look at gender also shows an inequitable use of resources in public schools. Heather J. Nicholson, the director of Girls Incorporated National Resource Center, discusses a research project in which she, along with others, "spent more than 700 hours observing girls in three communities across the United States . . . [and] found that girls face myriad obstacles to success." These obstacles include being "systematically if inadvertently deprived of . . . opportunities [to participate in science projects]; . . . a barrier of under-expectation"; too little "encouragement in math or science"; and "too few opportunities to learn how to be leaders" (1991). Again, discrepancies in treatment, access to resources, and opportunities are obstacles to achievement and thus to perceptions of intelligence. In such cases social forces may actually be eroding the "natural" capacities of children.

There is also a great deal of evidence that social practices can significantly enhance imagination and intelligence. A strong body of evidence indicates the influence of prenatal conditions on intelligence, and this research suggests a strong link between prenatal care and gestational development ("Prenatal Care" 1997). There are many other social factors that continue to affect intelligence, imagination, and learning from childhood into adulthood. For example, the school of critical pedagogy (a theory of education that critiques the power relations of mainstream pedagogy and seeks to empower students as active learners and critics) demonstrates the powerful influence of teaching on the creative, imaginative, and learning capacities of students, whether children or adults. Critical pedagogists assume that all students are capable of learning. One method for developing skills on this view is to engage students in critique, for example, of the educational system: how they may have been limited by it, and how they can respond constructively and politically to those limitations (hence the term "critical literacy").[11]

Imagination can best be understood not as a natural capacity which individuals happen to possess to varying degrees but as a dynamic relation between individuals and their social contexts. Twelve-step and other self-help programs demonstrate how many people are able to imagine and seek different ways of living through the support and example of others. Political movements such as feminism have altered the range of the imaginable by presenting new visions of human relations,[12] and many of those who have participated have experienced marked changes in behavior, feelings, and attitudes. And many who have come out as lesbian, gay, or bisexual, or participated in feminist consciousness-raising groups, attest that the sense of community they have gained has helped them overcome a sense of shame and enhance their self-respect; they discover that their "problems" are not personal flaws but arise from an oppressive social structure (O'Neill and Ritter 1992, Shreve 1989). In turn, a new vision is substituted: of women as active, intelligent, and capable; of heterosexual women as well as lesbians, bisexuals, and gay men as full persons rather than weak, deviant, or inferior. Such a vision of the self thus makes it possible to critique social hierarchies of gender or sexual orientation, and in turn to transform individual lives and broader social relations.

In addition, regardless of the origin of intelligence, imagination, or character (including moral development), many critics have argued that the very ideals by which these traits are measured are themselves based on the qualities favored or possessed by those in power.[13] Phyllis Teitelbaum argues that both the content and methodology of standardized testing manifest androcentric bias (1989).[14] Moreover, critics such as Harvard psychologist Howard Gardner argue that standard educational practices actually discourage the development of some forms of intelligence (Glazer 1994). Standardized testing and educational practices based on narrowly defined academic skills may disadvantage students whose talents have been hidden "whether by poverty, a different culture or learning delays and disabilities" (Glazer 1994, 14). Thus the very traits Gauthier considers most clearly "natural" in origin are themselves socially constituted, influenced by an individual's situation within a particular social context, and having a specific meaning and value relative to it. If environment plays the substantial role that I suggest, then not only is Gauthier mistaken in the assumption that they are ontological properties, but his understanding of the properties that constitute selfhood and how they do so is also called into question.

Perhaps it is not unreasonable to suggest, as Gauthier does, that one's health is more likely to fluctuate than one's major personality traits. Yet it is not as clear as Gauthier makes it that, in contrast to individual states of health, "character" traits and abilities are basically fixed and permanent, or that they spring from some inner essence, determined genetically or otherwise, and have meaning or value independent of particular social arrangements.

It is important to clarify at this point that I have engaged in this rather lengthy discussion of goods *other* than health for two reasons. First of all, Gauthier's arguments regarding access to health care are concerned with a tradeoff between health or health care and other kinds of goods. (This concern is also a central issue for other liberal theorists, although in my view the tradeoff is likely to be most pronounced in the work of those who are politically conservative.) Yet if, as I have argued, one's share of those goods considered natural is actually closely connected to one's share of other goods usually considered social, then the tradeoff is the product of a false dichotomy. A variety of examples supports the idea that this is in fact the case: ill health is clearly related to lack of prenatal care, low-paying jobs, inadequate housing and homelessness, poor nutrition, lack of access to family planning services, and other problems in families and communities.[15]

Second, I have discussed goods other than health at such length because they are the very ones Gauthier sees as uncontroversially natural in origin. If he has failed to recognize the ways in which "natural" goods are actually related to social causes, then it is important to examine critically his characterization of health as well.

Gauthier suggests several criteria for determining whether a trait is one that constitutes an individual: its origin (the degree to which it is chosen, socially conditioned, or innate), its duration, and its susceptibility to intervention. Diseases have an accidental, external origin—they "befall" a person. They are not willed (even though some individual choices, such as smoking, contribute), and thus in Gauthier's view do not reflect a person's character or identity, as do more voluntary aspects of their lives.

The application of these criteria is not always clear, however. Gauthier's conceptualization of the relation between health and identity seems to shift among three possibilities:

(1) Health is not among those traits that constitute individuality.

Gauthier distinguishes "between the status of an individual's condition of health and his or her abilities, interests, and traits of character. The latter we take to be constitutive of a particular individual" (1983, 184). The suggestion that health is not at all a constitutive trait is implicit, at the very least. Such an exclusion is plausible for Gauthier, given that his work exemplifies the most rationalist strand of liberal theory, valorizing rationality as the essence of personhood and conceptualizing agency as will, rational choice, and life plans.

Gauthier goes on to state that "such natural goods as intelligence, imagination, and industry . . . enter directly into individuality. . . . But a person's condition of health is not similarly constitutive of identity" (184). Are we to conclude that health is not constitutive at all, or is somehow constitutive in a different way from intelligence or imagination? The example Gauthier offers here is a "handicapped" person, who therefore "is thought of as something less than his or her real self" (184). I believe that this notion of the "real self" is slippery, and suggests that Gauthier's claims are not consistent. This gives rise to a second possibility:

(2) Only good health, or a certain minimum, is constitutive of a person's identity, while bad health is not.

One's "real self" for Gauthier is the self in good health, able-bodied. His discussion of this point, however, suggests further considerations which I believe undercut this interpretation as well.

While Gauthier views disease as "something that befalls a person, an accident in relation to nature or identity," he goes on to suggest that "the way in which we distinguish what is essential to a particular person from what accidentally befalls that person is affected by our beliefs about what is changeable through deliberate intervention, and so reflects a particular stage in the development of human technology" (184). He gives the example of "lepers, epileptics, and consumptives": now that treatments are available for these conditions, they do not enter into identity. This indeed is a comforting thought: not only does medicine physically heal, but it is also a kind of benevolent shepherd bringing ever more subjects into the fold of full agency or real personhood, transforming those who once were lepers into real persons.

But what of all those conditions that, despite the efficacy of the modern medical shepherd, are *still* incurable (for example, chronic diseases such as diabetes) or untreatable (such as some late-stage cancers)? Their existence suggests a third way of conceiving the relation of health to identity:

(3) Certain health conditions are among the traits constitutive of identity, while other health conditions are not: good health is constitutive, as are chronic and incurable conditions—those not susceptible to (medical) intervention.

This is not an alternative that Gauthier countenances; yet the example of formerly constitutive diseases such as leprosy only brings to mind the many conditions that, given the current state of medicine, are basically permanent, such as HIV infection, diabetes, and other chronic conditions or ongoing disabilities. Why are such cases not discussed? It seems clearly false to maintain that medical progress has for the most part done away with illnesses constitutive of identity, or that chronic illnesses are no longer experienced or perceived as constitutive, or perhaps that society has largely overcome its deep-seated prejudices against those with visible illnesses or disabilities.

Gauthier writes, "A person who is handicapped or impaired is thought of as something less than his or her real self—less than the self who would emerge were the handicap or impairment overcome" (184). Disability activists such as JoAnne Rome, however, express a very different perspective.[16] Born with a partial left arm, Rome struggles for self-acceptance in a world where sympathy and cruelty frequently accompany each other (1989). She is dismayed by the tone of a magazine article about a new prosthesis, billed as vastly superior to hooks or other prostheses such as the one she herself uses:

> The heading reads, "For children with missing limbs, myoelectric replacements offer a chance to lead LIVES THAT ARE WHOLE." . . . The article is laced with anecdotes and commentary from myo users, doctors and prosthetists who view the hook as obsolete. The emphasis is on how much like a real arm it is . . . how passing as two-handed makes life so much more comfortable for the wearer. . . . The medical establishment

promotes identification with the arm to the extent that the wearer is supposed to perceive her/his self as actually having two hands. (37–38)

While such devices certainly do facilitate increased functioning for many users, Rome points out who benefits most from the value of "normalcy" implicit in the description of the device: "These disabled kids [who testify to its benefits in the article] are asked to participate in a conspiracy that distorts reality and promotes a profound level of denial and self hate. . . . Built into the concept of prosthetics is the need of a fearful and cowardly world to avoid what is different and thus threatening to it. So we are compelled to cover up, to hide our 'defects' so that we are less offensive to others" (38). Rome describes a painful emotional process which finally leads her to conclude, "I am exactly what I'd been taught to deny" (39). In short, she does not perceive herself as less than her "real self"; she sees herself as a person — a person with a disability who deserves acceptance *as she is.*

Gauthier separates (ill) health conditions from identity, an ontological distinction that seems to offer hope to the person who wants to say, "I am not my disability," yet at the same time obscures the location of the disability in the social context. Much of the suffering that goes with disability is not random or accidental but entirely predictable, in at least two senses: first, through factors subject to human control which lead to injury, disease, or impairment; second, through resources and environments structured in accordance with the needs and purposes of only some people, in only some conditions.

In a novel by the disability activist Jean Stewart, the protagonist, Kate, writes to a friend dismayed by Kate's decision to equip herself with a wheelchair: "Nondisabled people seem obsessed with this moral principle that we should 'overcome' our disabilities, as if we live our whole lives locked in mortal combat with our bodies. As for me, I'm mostly content with mine, which is not to deny that I live a life of perpetual active combat, but rather to say that my body is the least of my adversaries" (1989, 240).

Kate finds that, as a woman with a disability, her greatest adversary is the array of disadvantages which social policies have created in some instances and failed to rectify in others. To take a parallel example from a different context, Timothy Murphy writes of so-called sexual reorientation therapy as "treating the person who suffers rather than stopping the forces that cause the suffering" (1992). Gauthier's metaphysical conception of disability as a characteristic of persons obscures the fact that disability involves not only bodily impairments but also (social) "forces that cause the suffering"— including medicine, which offers value judgments along with therapies.

I see Gauthier's metaphysical understanding of disability as based in part on a simplistic view of the relation between health and health care. For Gauthier, health seems to be on the order of an individual bank account into which nature makes an initial deposit, while health care is something like a foreign currency which, once exchanged, can be deposited directly into the same account. Although health care is not the same currency as health itself, and the rate of exchange may well vary between individuals, the two are nevertheless the same *kind* of good. This perception is extremely simplistic, completely overlooking rampant iatrogenic (caused by health care itself) and other socially occasioned illness, as well as the role of medicine in justifying and reinforcing social norms such as compulsory heterosexuality or femininity, and stigmatizing members of oppressed groups.

Gauthier's account of selfhood exhibits the bias that feminist theorists have long identified within philosophical liberalism: that despite defining human nature in terms of commonality and universality—the rationality presumed to be shared by all—traditional liberalism actually reflects the experiences of a privileged class. Feminist theorists argue that it is not coincidental that liberal philosophy, dominated by white heterosexual men of means, would generally conceptualize personhood in abstraction, identifying reason, the basis of choice, as human essence. Members of oppressed groups might find it more difficult to separate what is *unchosen* in themselves and their lives from their "real selves"—for it may be even harder to think of my "real self" as distinct from my gender "handicap," or the "handicap" of race or sexual orientation, than to understand a self distinct from its level of physical ability. Moreover, valorizing persons on the basis of commonality actually works against egalitarianism since those who differ from an implicit norm are thereby devalued.

Ultimately, measuring constitutive characteristics by their relative responsiveness to medical treatment is demeaning, especially for the disabled. If a disabled person is "less than his or her real self," not only must she deal with bodily imperfections, but she has become an imperfect *person* as well.

Far from advancing the egalitarian goal of valuing each individual alike, based on the capacity for rationality shared by moral agents, such a view actually perpetuates an "ableist" social standard; indeed, it diminishes the status of people with disabilities as rational agents by linking "real selfhood" to a certain level of physical ability. What is more, locating the lack of the "self" in the disabled person obscures the social causes of suffering by portraying disability as a combat between reason and the body rather than between a person and a frequently punishing social environment.

Daniels and Access to Health Care

In *Just Health Care* (1985), Norman Daniels provides an account of access to health care which he sees as compatible with the overall outlook of Rawls's *A Theory of Justice*.[17] Rawls and Daniels share with Gauthier certain assumptions of philosophical liberalism, yet they advocate politically liberal views, believing that certain kinds of unjust disadvantages occur frequently in society. Daniels attempts to rectify such disadvantage in the context of health care. But though his work has strong advantages over Gauthier's, Daniels too relies on a simplistic boundary between the natural and the social, uncritically takes aspects of the existing health care system for granted, and significantly underestimates the importance of social group differentials, thereby failing to address the problem of oppression and undermining the effort to address "disadvantage."

Because of the particular attributes of health care, according to Daniels, just distribution requires special considerations. First, health care can help to compensate some less fortunate individuals for physiological disadvantages due to the circumstances of their birth which strongly affect their life prospects. Second, Daniels notes, "Impairments of natural species functioning reduce the range of opportunity open to the individual in which he may construct his 'plan of life' or conception of the good" (1985, 27)— a pluralistic appeal to individual choice which is characteristic of liberalism. Since health care in many cases can prevent or overcome the constraints on opportunity caused by health problems, and since the distribution of health care is a matter of public policy, Daniels argues that decisions of access must be based on the special relationship of health care to opportunity.

Daniels's relation of opportunity to justice is heavily influenced by Rawls's concept of "fair equality of opportunity" (1971), a tool for evaluating the fairness of competitions on a procedural basis. Following Rawls, Daniels argues that "talents and skills" rather than "morally irrelevant features [such as] race, religion, ethnic origin, sex" must determine the distribution of positions (Daniels 1985, 39–40). Daniels shares Rawls's view that fair equality of opportunity does not entail equality of outcome. Rawls argues that while the welfare of everyone, including the untalented and unskilled, must be taken into account in the distribution of assets, justice does not require equality of outcome if, for example, rewarding the most productive members of society with a greater share would result in a greater overall level of benefits for all those who are least well off.

Daniels departs from Rawls by conceptualizing opportunity more broadly than the latter, who emphasizes jobs and careers. Daniels conceives of opportunity as relative to particular societies, introducing the concept of "normal opportunity range," which "for a given society is the array of life plans reasonable persons in it are likely to construct for themselves" (33). Furthermore, "the share of the normal range open to an individual is . . . determined in a fundamental way by his talents and skills. Fair equality of opportunity does not require opportunity to be equal for all persons. It requires only that it be equal for persons with similar skills and talents" (33).

Daniels's concept of "normal opportunity range" recognizes that the vicissitudes of human physicality can interfere with opportunity. In addition, to correct for what he sees as Rawls's overly narrow focus on jobs and careers, Daniels introduces an *age-relative* opportunity range: "Life plans, we might note, clearly have stages, which reflect important divisions in the life cycle" (104). Thus, an important task for justice is the "attempt to assure individuals a fair chance at enjoyment of the normal opportunity range for each life-stage" (104).

Daniels maintains, furthermore, that "impairment of normal functioning through disease and disability restricts an individual's opportunity relative to that portion of the normal range his skills and talents would have made available to him were he healthy" (33–34). Health care itself, as a basic social institution, is given the job of ensuring egalitarian opportunity: "From the perspective of justice . . . the moral function of the health-care system must be to help guarantee fair equality of opportunity" (41). (Recall that Gauthier, in contrast, focuses initially on health itself as a primary good, and goes on from there to develop a view of just access to health care.)

Ultimately, Daniels intends the concept of "impairment of the normal opportunity range" to be used "as a fairly crude measure of the relative importance of health-care needs at the macro level" (35). For Daniels, the most important advantage of this account is the fact that it captures a social guarantee of access to care as an obligation of justice.

Unlike Gauthier, who argues for a very limited view of social obligations regarding health care distribution, Daniels provides grounds for a much more extensive set of obligations, at least in part because of his desire to improve conditions for those who are worst off. He is extremely concerned with ameliorating the unfair disadvantage faced by some individuals as a result of their starting points in life, and shows that the general fact of disadvantage exacerbates problems of access in specific situations. For example, in a chapter on the question of rationing health care on the basis of age, he notes that many elderly people are disadvantaged in a variety of ways, not only through experiences and circumstances directly related to their age, but also because age may magnify and complicate earlier experiences of disadvantage. He also provides strong grounds for treating health care as one of the basic social institutions that should satisfy principles of justice, based on the convincing argument that health care problems are related to justice in terms of the constraints they can impose on opportunity. This deep concern for human suffering and the moral and political urgency of rectifying it make his work far more amenable to the concerns of activist health movements than Gauthier's.

Nonetheless, it is noteworthy that Daniels's theory shares certain significant weaknesses with Gauthier's, despite the two theorists' political differences. The relation Daniels draws between health and opportunity is indicative of a larger problem. While health problems can undermine opportunity, constraints on opportunity can certainly undermine health as well. This omission points to a significant failing: Daniels's emphasis on disadvantage blocks recognizing and analyzing the more pervasive and systematic phenomenon of oppression. He does not recognize the complex interconnections of various harms which reinforce one another, working together to constrain members of a particular group on a differential ba-

sis. Despite his concern for rectifying disadvantage, Daniels treats these issues as a problem that happens to befall members of a group. A multifactorial analysis of oppression, by contrast, addresses the problem much more
clearly in terms of the mutually reinforcing effects of multiple aspects of
oppression.

Take, for example, the case of lesbian, bisexual, and gay people. Heterosexism interferes with our health and limits our opportunity at the same
time—phenomena that are not distinct but strongly related. The psychological stresses of heterosexist oppression have profound consequences,
physical as well as emotional, and may influence our sense of the efficacy
and value of necessary self-care and risk avoidance. Limited opportunities
in turn may restrict access to health insurance and other resources which
strongly affect health. On a larger scale, as we saw in earlier chapters, heterosexism structures research design and clinical practice, and can shape
providers' attitudes and institutional policies, leading to problems in health
care itself. Both overt and more subtle discrimination, as well as the internalized pressure which gay people may feel to keep their lives and identities secret from employers and co-workers, can limit opportunity—not
merely in the narrow external sense, but in the deeper sense of life plans and
expectations as well (O'Neill and Ritter 1992). The relation between health
and opportunity is clearly a very complex one whose social significance
cannot fully be understood without a multifactorial analysis of oppression.
The abstract procedural emphasis of the fair equality of opportunity approach simply offers no guidance in addressing these issues of social group
differentials which must be structured into the moral evaluation of social
policy.

Daniels addresses other important issues in ways that fail to expose underlying problems, and thus seriously limits the ability to rectify them. For
example, his understanding of disability as socially constituted to some degree—or "society-relative," as he puts it—while far more useful than Gauthier's, is not adequate. Dyslexia, he points out, would not be a significant
impairment in a nonliterate society: "Thus the social importance of particular diseases is a notion which we ought to view as socially relative"
(34). Here he appropriately acknowledges the embeddedness of particular forms of disability within specific social contexts without attributing to
them some kind of ontological status. Despite this useful impetus toward

a "society-relative" account, however, Daniels, too, seems simply to assume a clear boundary between the natural and the social. A crucial insight of a material-semiotic understanding is to view health and health problems as always embedded within specific social contexts rather than as ontological properties of individuals. Such a view makes it possible not only to evaluate individual health, pathologizing individuals' states and prescribing individual cures, but also to evaluate the social contexts in which these problems arise, diagnosing and transforming those social forces that may be implicated in the suffering rather than restricting attention to the sufferer alone. Although Daniels does recognize that dyslexia, for example, exists in relation to a particular context, he does not recognize the moral necessity of evaluating those social forces that constitute individual impairments in specific contexts, not just the impairments themselves.

Daniels also treats the capacities, skills, and talents of individuals as basically innate or natural properties—much as Gauthier does—although he recognizes an additional layer of social influence: "Skills and talents can be undeveloped or misdeveloped because of social conditions" (34). This recognition is valuable, of course, because it leads Daniels to argue for the importance of providing a certain level of both education and health care where necessary to help individuals enjoy their portion of the normal opportunity range. Nonetheless, he takes for granted some baseline ontological differences in the capacities of individuals. I have argued earlier in this chapter that individual shares of talents and skills (specifically intelligence and imagination) are quite susceptible to various social influences, and that standards intended to measure them often reflect the interests of those who are already advantaged. Building these baseline differences between individuals into a theory of justice in health care simply excludes pressing social problems from the domain of justice altogether.

Inadvertently, additional problems are taken for granted as well. Both Daniels and Gauthier provide an account of the requirements of justice regarding the design of the health care system. Neither one, however, questions some important basic features of the current system, including most of those I addressed in the context of women's health and HIV.[18] Of those examples, their respective frameworks would generally include only those problems directly related to access, leaving many untouched, such as social relations within the health care system, and the deeper issues of the medical pathologizing of certain groups, as well as the cultural authority of medicine.[19]

In short, the conception of justice relied on by these authors, which consists entirely of fair distribution, excludes vitally important aspects of health and health care. Iris Young (1990) correctly notes that justice in regard to health has been construed in terms of access to care, owing to the distributive paradigm which is central to liberal theory. She argues that this paradigm leaves out issues that cannot be conceived in terms of goods that can be allocated and distributed. In the previous chapters I have illustrated and defended this thesis in the case of medicine: the distributive paradigm has no direct means of addressing the pathologization of women and of gay and bisexual men, or of the underlying authority of medicine, a problem I take to exemplify the larger failure to conceptualize oppression as a central aspect of justice in health.

Finally, I consider Daniels's view of personhood useful in being at least apparently less rationalist in some ways than Gauthier's, yet I wonder why this view does not result in a more thoroughgoing analysis of the medical system. Daniels is always concerned with the array of material needs entailed by human physicality; for example, he includes the basic means of survival, such as food ("adequate nutrition") and shelter, in the category of legitimate health care needs (32). Although Gauthier is hardly unaware of human physicality, Daniels gives it a much more prominent role, recognizing the moral significance of material conditions and related human needs.

Despite this less rationalist view of personhood, however, there is a related aspect of health that has no place in Daniels's account: the subjective experience of health and health care and its implications for justice. The women's health and AIDS movements identify this as a key issue, given the many problems in the treatment of women and gay and bisexual men in the health care system. Daniels expresses interest in the impact of health care on self-respect, but he does not address this topic at any length and does not see it as directly related to justice (71). Rawls, however, considers self-respect "perhaps the most important primary good" (1971, 440), although he does not spell out the practical implications of this conviction. But the recognition, though it may be difficult to integrate with the rationalist values of liberal theory, is extremely important. While not all liberal theorists would necessarily deny that health is valuable in and of itself, the liberal identification of human nature in terms of reason, will, and choice leaves little room to integrate the subjective experience of embodiment (as well as other nonrational aspects of subjectivity) into the conception of justice—a topic I will address further.

Liberal theories of access to health care as exemplified by Daniels and Gauthier are all linked to the rationalist conception of choice and its relation to the social context. From this perspective, choice (or "rational choice," as it is often termed) is understood in the abstract as a human faculty arising from reason rather than a dynamic relation between individual consciousness and a particular socially constituted set of alternatives.[20]

I turn next to Robert Dickman's work, which represents an alternative to other liberal theorists' avoidance of the topic of social relations within the health care system and their impact on self-respect. He also makes the idea of "choice" much less abstract in at least one sense, by focusing on the choice (or lack thereof) of health care providers by low-income patients. He addresses the subjective aspects of health care as an important concern for justice, an approach with the potential to further the goal of accommodating the needs of the disempowered. In Dickman's theory, as in Daniels's and Gauthier's, the conceptualization of choice plays an important role in the conclusions about access to health care.

Dickman and the Subjective Aspects of Health Care

Robert Dickman's "Operationalizing Respect for Persons" (1983) is a notable exception to the dominant access-oriented treatment of justice and health care. Dickman focuses on nontechnical and subjective aspects of health care (that is, qualitative aspects other than competence or efficacy of care) which are not usually addressed by theorists working within the distributive paradigm, although he indirectly acknowledges that distributive concerns are relevant to his argument (presupposing some degree of willingness on the part of society to provide or subsidize care for those who cannot afford it). Instead, situating his argument in the context of the health care that is usually available to the urban poor, he argues that certain aspects of this care tend to exacerbate drastically the loss of autonomy and self-respect associated with illness. Because of their economic circumstances, the urban poor have only two options: to endure assaults on their self-respect when they are already made vulnerable by illness, or to forgo needed care. Dickman believes that this situation is inconsistent with the obligation to treat all persons with respect. Thus he argues that justice demands certain qualitative changes in the subjective experience of health care by the urban poor, and proposes a method for evaluating specific health care settings according to the principle of respect for persons.

He identifies two features of care at large urban public health clinics: environmental problems and lack of continuity in the care of individuals. The former include a "lack of nonmedical amenities"—no appointment systems, long waiting times (Dickman mentions a study that found "an average wait of over three hours for a physician encounter of about 7½ minutes")—as well as impatient and judgmental attitudes on the part of professionals, and repetition of procedures such as pelvic exams during a single visit for the benefit of medical students in training (167). In regard to the second category, he finds that "patients in this system fail to develop a continuing and meaningful relationship with a single health care provider," particularly when they are hospitalized (167). These problems, Dickman claims, affect "the way people (both consumers and providers) are made to *feel* within that setting" (168–69). Thus, "the fundamental deficiency of that system lies in its failure to respect the autonomy of its clients and to create an atmosphere that allows them to maintain their self-respect" (169).

Dickman bases his argument not only on the kind of treatment low-income patients receive, but also on what he sees as an "essential ontological assault produced by illness or injury" prior to treatment (169). It is this aspect of illness and injury that leads Dickman to distinguish health care from other goods. He argues: "The fact of being ill poses the greatest threat to the integrity and freedom of any individual. Ill or injured patients . . . become constantly preoccupied with their health problems. This preoccupation, along with pain and/or suffering, prevents them from making unencumbered choices about important aspects of their lives" (169). For Dickman, then, health care is unique because of the need to ameliorate the erosion of agency and free will imposed by illness, which he sees as the most significant interference with these capacities and values which humans can experience.

He therefore concludes that when health care has diminished "the already seriously threatened autonomy of the patient . . . by the very nature of the delivery system, a moral violation can be perceived to exist" (169). This violation occurs in two ways. First, because public clinic care is generally perceived as "charity," clients may lose self-respect and autonomy. Student providers may approach this work primarily as part of their training; if so, they "will be less capable of acknowledging the rights of their clients," while those providers "who view their work with clinic patients as beneficent will at best be paternalistic in regard to their interactions with them" (170). Second, the environment of the clinic itself "makes it difficult or impossible for professionals to act in ways that show respect for persons" (170).

According to Dickman, invoking the principle of respect and calling on providers to abide by it would be an important and morally binding step, yet "not sufficient to bring about reform within the system" (173). He proposes evaluating a system on the basis of its acceptability to "reasonable judges" who have other options available to them for care. His concept of the reasonable judge excludes "those whose personal freedoms have been stripped away in so many other ways that further encroachments, as within the health care setting, will not be accurately perceived" (174). He emphasizes that he makes this exclusion not because he sees the disadvantaged as "incapable of knowing when violations to their dignity have taken place," but because, "since no other options may be open to them or they may have become 'immune' to these encroachments, their continued use of the service may not *in and of itself* be convincing proof of the adequacy of the service" (175).

To evaluate by this method would require "a pluralistic system of health care with the existence of alternative and morally viable options," which Dickman thinks is in fact the case in the United States (175). Furthermore, he says, we can imagine a system that retains clients who have other options, yet treats some of its clients with respect but not others. He argues, however, that "changes in the system designed to pass the test will clearly be applicable to all. . . . An atmosphere that satisfies the reasonable judge is more likely than not to spill over to all involved" (176). Dickman concludes that in all health care encounters, "there would be at least two necessary components of a decent minimum" right to health care: "a continuous relationship with a competent provider and . . . an environment that does not allow for loss of respect" (180).

In summary, the central tenets of Dickman's argument are that illness inherently injures a person's autonomy, integrity, and self-respect; that certain subjectively unpleasant features of health care for low-income patients are incompatible with respectful treatment and thus compound the problems of illness; and that the remedy for this problem is a procedure that would measure the subjective satisfaction of "reasonable judges" who use a particular health care service.

Dickman's work has significant advantages. Unlike Daniels or Gauthier, Dickman actually reflects on the social relations that occur within the health care system. In arguing that certain aspects of these social relations must be transformed because they erode the self-respect of already disadvantaged people, he addresses an important concern which theorists of the distributive paradigm tend to neglect (probably because of the nature of the paradigm itself); these insights are critically needed, and his proposed remedy seems likely to benefit the urban poor significantly. Yet this work too fails to grapple adequately with social group differentials.

First of all, there are several ways in which Dickman also takes for granted that firm boundary between the natural and the social which should be examined more critically as an aspect of the moral analysis of social relations. Even though Dickman illuminates the ethical significance of social relations within the health care setting, his approach removes health care from its interactions with other aspects of the social structure. The treatment of illness as ontological assault removes the interactions of health care and society from ethical analysis. Moreover, respect for persons requires attending to differences, such as those of race, culture, ethnicity, economic class, and gender. Together these considerations reveal serious limitations in Dickman's notion of the reasonable judge, and they suggest that the standard distinction between "disease" and "illness" (the former indicating the clinical, biochemical condition, and the latter the individual experience of that condition within a life context) is to some extent based on a false dichotomizing of subjectivity and objectivity, which inappropriately severs subjective aspects of care from clinical aspects and from the understanding of access itself.

I find Dickman's treatment of illness and injury as "ontological assault" overly simplistic. Although many serious illnesses and injuries clearly do constitute a fundamental assault on the personhood of individuals, some maladies for which clients seek medical treatment do not. Dickman states, "The fact of being ill poses *the* greatest threat to the integrity and freedom of any individual" (169; emphasis added). Not only does Dickman assume the ontological status of all illness, but also he neglects the possibility of *external* threats to integrity and freedom which are equal or comparable in scope to those posed by illness. Most likely, illness constitutes the greatest threat only to the relatively privileged. Many disability activists attest to external circumstances which they find at least as disempowering as their own physical states. Recall the comments of disability activists Jean Stewart and JoAnne Rome, who have adapted to the conditions of their bodies but find the struggle to adjust to social conditions far more difficult. Consider also the pervasive violence against members of oppressed groups, where hatred, sexual contempt, and physical brutality create a climate of fear which threatens those who are not physically assaulted along with those who are. One's very mobility may be constrained in order to avoid potentially dangerous situations. Restrictive and otherwise harmful social conditions may impose threats to integrity and freedom which sometimes overshadow those imposed by illness; thus, not only is illness socially constituted, but so are differentials in degrees of personal freedom and autonomy.

Another aspect of Dickman's position which prevents the analysis of important issues of justice in health care is its retention of the abstract individualism of liberal theory. His "reasonable judge" standard employs the abstract or generic human conception, which has been criticized extensively. Considering the possible objection to his argument that reasonable judges might be satisfied with the care that they receive, while other clients at the same facility might not be treated with the same respect, he notes: "Changes in the system designed to pass the test will clearly be applicable to all [clients]. . . . [W]orkers in this system will not be constantly 'shifting gears' depending on the particular client. . . . An atmosphere that satisfies the reasonable judge is more likely than not to spill over to all involved" (176). This statement completely overlooks the significance of difference.

While some changes that please any particular "reasonable judge" would undoubtedly prove to be generally satisfying, not every behavior or policy will generalize equally to everyone. Persons are not generic containers of reason, but have beliefs, needs, and preferences formed in the context of specific social positions and identities. Moreover, our treatment of others is affected by our perceptions of difference—perceptions that do not occur in a social vacuum.

Recall the discussion of cultural imperialism early in this chapter, a phenomenon that includes the perceptual habit of generalizing the standards, beliefs, or preferences of dominant groups onto members of oppressed groups in disempowering ways. Cheryl Killion, an African American nurse, reports a white head-nurse's misinterpretation of an African American patient:

> One time the head nurse called a special case conference to discuss an African-American mother who had called her newborn infant "bad." It was the head nurse's contention that this mother had a problem in bonding with her newborn and might abuse the baby. However, the head nurse had not observed the body language of the mother nor did she understand the full meaning of "bad." The mother was actually bonding wonderfully with her new son. She held him often, talked to him in a soothing voice, handled him gently and breastfed him without difficulty. It was clear to me that she was a loving, attentive, proud mother. . . . [To] her, "Oh, he's so-o ba-ad!" meant that he was alert, active and smart. After I provided this explanation to the staff, the mother was spared a visit from the staff psychiatrist and a social service follow-up. (1990, 246)

The head nurse's interpretation of the mother's interaction with her infant serves as a clear example of cultural imperialism, in which "gear-shifting," or treating various clients differently, occurs so smoothly as to be unconscious on the part of the staff, despite Dickman's claim that "gear-shifting" will not occur in a system that offers basic care and a certain level of important "amenities." It seems quite unlikely that the satisfaction of a white "reasonable judge," whether male or female, would necessarily represent the experience of this new mother.

One might ask why this is an example of gear-shifting, if the head nurse would be concerned with any parent who called her newborn "bad." Her reaction to this language, however—a reaction which is itself based on "standard English" linguistic norms coded as white—is not the only problem. A closer analysis suggests the white head nurse's underlying and possibly unconscious suspicion of an African American patient. In addition to forming an inappropriate and potentially punitive judgment based on a single word, she failed to notice other cues, such as the mother's gentleness and warmth with her child, which were obvious to another nurse. I suspect that she would have been less oblivious to these qualities had her patient been white. This incident indicates just how smoothly gears can be shifted, perhaps even in the absence of conscious negative intentions.

The problem with the reasonable judge standard is not only the possibility of ethnocentric racism or cultural imperialism but also its inadequacy for addressing issues of economic class. Even the issue of what constitutes access itself, and what constitutes barriers to access, is not the same for all groups. I bring this issue up here because I contend that so-called basic access and subjective satisfaction are not necessarily the separate issues they are usually taken to be.

The standard model for delivering health care to the urban poor is by means of large centralized sites, a model that has been criticized as being located and arranged for the convenience of professional staff rather than patients, and not merely being ineffective in meeting patient needs but actually imposing difficult and unnecessary burdens on them. These include some of the problems Dickman mentions, as well as external factors in the community which impinge on the accessibility of care: living and working conditions, transportation, child care, and other such issues. People may be forced to choose between earning a day's wages and obtaining needed medical services, while others miss appointments because of problems with transportation or child care. Newer models of community-based care offer alternatives such as small neighborhood-based clinics rather than large centralized facilities, extended hours of service, and outreach, taking preventive health care out into the community, to schools, church programs, PTA meetings, and other forums.[21]

This newer model, incorporating considerations beyond the limits of the distributive paradigm (which conceives of barriers to access in essentially financial terms), addresses Dickman's concerns with certain subjective aspects of care and adds a new level of cultural and community specificity to the abstraction of Dickman's liberal framework. First, treating patients in a particular community with respect requires awareness of the values and culture of specific groups within that community. Second, it requires awareness of conditions within the health care setting which might be perfectly satisfactory to some clients yet not so for others. More subtle factors affecting satisfaction with care, and on an even more basic level accessibility itself, are the hours, location, and settings in which care is delivered. Meeting basic needs, particularly in urban locations, requires the services of translators, social workers, and outreach staff as part of the health care team. It is essential to address all those external factors that impinge on both access and satisfaction: transportation, child care, local employers' labor policies, as well as living and working conditions that can promote or hinder the efficacy of care.

The Women and Children with AIDS Program at Cook County Hospital in Chicago exemplifies a public hospital program designed in response to a specific constituency's needs. Physician Mardge Cohen, one of the creators of the program as well as its director, notes: "All over the city we could see a growing concentration of services for gay men and [male] IV drug users who were HIV positive—but nothing for women. AIDS was [understood] first and foremost [as] a men's disease" (quoted in McClory 1991). The program Cohen helped to develop in response to this urgent need provides medical care for women and children at the same site as well as comprehensive support services, including "professional counseling, especially for chronic problems such as alcohol and drug abuse that may go along with AIDS[,] . . . case managers to help women get the medical care and financial aid they're entitled to, . . . health education, legal advice, child care, and peer support groups" (McClory 1991).

In *The Invisible Epidemic,* Gena Corea explains the services offered by the same program and its objectives. Along with child care and meals for the women, group support is considered essential:

> From the beginning, a support group was part of the standard of care at County. It should be everywhere, Cohen maintained, because the women live in a terrible, debilitating isolation, unable to talk with anyone else about what they are going through. . . .

The facilitators came to name what happened in the group "the evolution of dignity." The women were expected to sit for hours with ill
children in the packed waiting rooms of large and unresponsive institutions. In the group, the women . . . modeled for each other assertive behavior in getting aid, entitlements, child care, and in dealing with Cook
County Hospital itself. (1992, 156–57)

The support group is not merely an additional service which benefits the
members but an important source of information for providers: "The support group gave the health team feedback on what issues the women were
facing, medically and socially, so that the providers could figure out which
programs could be discontinued, which should go on, what needed to be
created" (157). Group members also make an important contribution
to the community through prevention efforts: "Interested women in the
group were trained as paid peer HIV-prevention educators in a six-week
program. They then went out and talked about HIV in various community settings" (157).

Cohen sees all aspects of the program as integral parts of health care for
women with AIDS. Innovative approaches were necessary, first of all, to
address basic medical needs, given the medical neglect of women in the
context of HIV. In addition, the needs and concerns of the women in their
social roles as women and mothers had to be addressed, along with drug
and alcohol issues, the negotiation of condom use and other aspects of risk
reduction, and a host of other psychosocial issues. Cohen understands all
of these "nonmedical" concerns as having a profound impact on the manifestations and progression of HIV in her women and children patients, and
in order to address these problems, the program had to be designed and
modified on the basis of their day-to-day needs and concerns. Thus, the importance of a "nonmedical" service, the peer support group, lies not only
in its psychotherapeutic value for patients but also in its role as a necessary
source of information for the "experts" who must understand the psychosocial, gendered components of HIV as part of the "medical" picture.

One may object at this point (both to Dickman's argument and my critique of it) that when health care is available to the urban poor, as long as
that care is medically competent (even if subjectively unsatisfying), at least
the important basic needs have been satisfied. But this intuition is a mis-

leading product of the distributive paradigm, based on an assumption that the main barrier to decent care is financial. Although Dickman does go beyond certain limits of this paradigm in his introduction of subjective concerns, he nonetheless poses an inappropriately rigid dichotomy between the subjective versus the narrowly medical (hence supposedly "objective") aspects of care, a formulation that undercuts the ability of his "reasonable judge" standard to address the needs of the disempowered.

This point can be illustrated in the context of the standard distinction between "disease" (in reference to biochemical states, for which medical treatment may be sought) and "illness" (understood as the experience of a particular person living with a certain disease). Recall my discussion in the previous chapter of the Flexnerian model of medicine, as defended by Donald Seldin, in which medicine is strictly concerned with the treatment of diseases, and not with illness or lived experience. The physician's relationship to illness is relatively insignificant, perceived in terms of "bedside manner," not medicine "itself." Dickman's distinction between medical care and amenities fits neatly into this dichotomy: "amenities" are not part of the basic care necessary for the biomedical treatment of disease, but features of the medical interaction which may affect the lived experience of the patient beyond the biochemical states as such. Yet I would argue not only that this distinction is based on an unnecessarily dualistic separation of body and mind, but also that it is simply not as accurate as it may intuitively seem.

Researchers and clinicians in the growing field of mind-body medicine, or psychoneuroimmunology, challenge the separation of subjective and personal aspects of "illness" from the clinical entity of disease states in a particular patient. Treating disease adequately requires the clinician to understand and address what an illness means in the lives of patients and their families. For example, Ron Anderson, M.D. (chairman of the board of the Texas Department of Health, and chief executive officer of the innovative Parkland Hospital), mentions the example of two patients who have suffered heart attacks, a truck driver and a banker. The clinical manifestations of coronary disease are comparable in these patients, yet affect each life in dramatically different ways in terms of financial repercussions, family concerns, employability and rehabilitation, and ways of coping with loss and fear. The truck driver most likely will become unemployed, while the banker enjoys various advantages as a result of his socioeconomic status which provide some insulation from the problems of coronary disease. Anderson argues that adequate medical practice requires one to understand as far as possible the life contexts and subjective experiences of each person in order to treat the disease, by addressing, for example, the potential health risks to the truck driver of chronic stress due to unemployment (Moyers 1993, 28–29). Doing so would entail not only incorporating information from the patient's subjective perspective into the medical knowledge base, but also addressing the subjective states of patients, their fears and anxieties, their preferences and life plans, in the context of medical care itself.

Despite Dickman's concern for the urban poor, his conception of the "reasonable judge" standard overlooks social difference as one of the constitutive aspects of illness and a factor that shapes the experience of health care as well, as we have seen in the contexts of ethnocentric racism, economic class, and the gender aspects of HIV. It is both the abstraction of Dickman's "reasonable judge" standard which is problematic in this regard and its individualism as well. I do not mean to suggest that Dickman is wrong to be concerned with the mistreatment of individuals as such, or that he should instead be concerned with something else altogether, such as the status of groups. Rather, I think that the two should not be separated. Dickman focuses on the lack of respect experienced by clinic patients as individuals. Killion's story, along with other examples I have cited, suggests that treating people with respect or treating them justly requires understanding people as members of social groups as well as unique individuals. Doing so would require not just an acknowledgment of difference, cultural or otherwise, but also an analysis of oppressive forces in society and how they affect members of specific groups. Given the extent of oppression in our society, treating people with respect entails not merely granting them respect as *individuals* but actually transforming social relations so that oppressed *groups* can occupy places of respect in the social structure.

Such an analysis would reveal the connection between specific practices such as social relations within the health care setting and those in the society at large. Dickman's silence on these broader concerns (which I have argued are directly relevant) reveals the assumption that the two realms are separate, or at least that ethical analysis of health care need not address their connection.

Is the "reasonable judge" approach at all viable, given these criticisms? Could the problems with its abstract individualism which I have outlined be remedied? We might, for example, consider the satisfaction of a panel of judges, with a demographic makeup reflecting the composition of the body of clients who use a certain facility: persons of diverse races and ethnicities, classes, sexual orientations, family situations, life stages and life plans; women and men; people with diverse disabilities as well as those who are not currently disabled.[22]

Such an attempt may be an important step toward Dickman's goal of meeting the health care needs of the disempowered. Yet this modification alone leaves too many problems unanswered, such as the question of who gets sick and why, and the harmful aspects of medical concepts and practices. It is not enough to identify the organization of the clinic, its "lack of amenities," and the behavior of individuals within that environment as problematic; it is also necessary to question medical authority and its relation to other social practices that affect the disempowered.

4

Restricted Choices: The Social Constitution of Health Care Needs

The experience of illness often contains an existential dimension of incoherence; it is senseless, imposed arbitrarily by fate. Consider "affliction," a biblical word which brings to mind the travails of Job, whose suffering was random, morally arbitrary: he did not deserve it. This notion captures an important aspect of illness. It speaks, for example, to those whose lives, indeed their sense of the world and their place in it, have been ruptured beyond repair by AIDS, as well as to those who have invented from the epidemic a new sense of purpose for themselves.[1]

In another respect, however, illness is not always so senseless. Much of it is entirely coherent, even predictable, through its links to social contexts that interfere with health. Yet the sense of sickness as ill-fated departure from ordinary human experience exerts subtle but far-reaching influence in bioethics. Both aspects of this general outlook are problematic. Conceiving illness, suffering, and physical frailty mainly in opposition to ordinary experience assumes a standpoint best understood as one of privilege, in contrast to the stance of those for whom these conditions *are* in some sense ordinary experience (as illustrated in Chapter 3 by disability). Furthermore, although sickness is indeed morally arbitrary in that it is undeserved, it is not entirely random, given the multiple factors contributing to social group differentials in health and illness. The knowledge that illness is (undeserved) affliction seems to have spread to tacit assumptions of its randomness.

The framework of liberalism often tends to replicate this "affliction" view of illness, and of health care needs as well, in abstraction from the social world. In efforts to preserve their belief in an equal ability of everyone to make life choices, liberal theorists often overlook the material circumstances that constrain these choices for oppressed groups, and that strongly influence their physical and emotional health and well-being. This problem exemplifies the need to abandon the "natural" versus "social" dichotomy of human experience in favor of a material-semiotic understanding of health and illness, which recognizes the inseparability of the two.

A particular view of health—what it is, and how it is related to the social world—is the basis for any theory of health care needs. In turn, a theory of health care access hinges on the understanding of health care needs: what counts as a legitimate need depends on what health is, and what enhances or undermines it. Norman Daniels and David Gauthier, like many other liberal theorists, rely on an empirical or "descriptive" account of health. My contention, however, is that a material-semiotic understanding of health and health care needs is necessary to avoid reproducing the sexist, heterosexist, and erotophobic influences of medicine which I have criticized in previous chapters; and that neither the distributive paradigm of justice nor the descriptive account of health offers the means to detect or to remedy the problem. Ultimately, this suggests that the descriptive account should be abandoned in favor of an explicitly anti-oppression framework of health and health care needs. I first assess these theories of health care needs and the descriptive account that grounds them, then examine issues in women's health that raise challenges for these views.

Gauthier's "Affliction" Concept of Health Care Needs

For Gauthier, the unequal need for care is the main ethical problem in the arena of health. He chooses to restrict his arguments to the question of "access to health care . . . where the need is not socially occasioned," as opposed to cases in which "the need for such care may be attributed to some specific public or private activity" (1983, 182). He identifies three categories of "socially occasioned" diseases: those that are "occupationally based" (such as "exposure to radioactive materials"), those resulting from personal habits (such as lung cancer among smokers), and those that are the result of "measures intended to eliminate other deviations" (such as "allergic responses to penicillin") (180). In the paragraph and a half that Gauthier devotes to this topic, he states, "Some of these activities, such as smoking, may be viewed as entirely discretionary; care for ill effects may then appropriately be the individual's expense" (181). By contrast, "care for occupation-related diseases should be legally required to be assumed by the employer, over and above standard wages and benefits" (181). If this expense is too great for the employer to bear, then, in Gauthier's view, "the total social costs of the activity exceed the total social benefits" (181–82).

Beyond grounding health care needs in the descriptive account of health, Gauthier does not specify their characteristics, which suggests that he understands this account to entail a straightforward and self-evident conception of health care needs as well. Gauthier argues, "The moral significance of health care needs is . . . to be found . . . in the idea of natural and normal human functioning, which is a core part of our conception of a good human life" (184). Finally, he concludes: "Access to health care should reflect an impartial concern with the various deviations from natural human functioning that, through no fault of either the individual or society, actually impede the good lives persons might otherwise expect through social cooperation based on individual talents, aptitudes, and interests" (201).

Gauthier's view of "socially occasioned" health care needs is highly problematic, and not only because it is a cursory discussion. First of all, in arguing that the costs of health care needs in this category should be borne by those carrying out the activity that gave rise to those needs, Gauthier seems to understand cost only in the very narrow sense of dollars spent on treatments and services. Yet living with an illness imposes costs or burdens far beyond the dollars spent on care. Gauthier does not discuss the costs, for example, borne by workers exposed to radiation and by their families; they are living with cancer whether or not their medical expenses are paid. Such costs to individual health, and the psychological and secondary economic costs to themselves and their families, constitute a very serious harm which Gauthier completely overlooks.

He seems to assume that it is permissible for one party (in his example, private business interests, which for some reason he includes under the rubric of "public") to benefit at the expense of other individuals' health, as long as the responsible party pays the medical expenses. Gauthier considers only two questions: whether the burden of these expenses is assigned fairly, and whether for a particular "public activity" the practice will be cost-effective, given the medical expense entailed. He overlooks other concerns, such as the value of bodily integrity, which surely requires very significant considerations to override it; and the fact that those most likely to face serious occupational and environmental health risks are the working class and the urban poor, particularly people of color—groups whose life prospects are already diminished in comparison to others'.[2]

In general, Gauthier's notions of cost and benefit, and of responsibility for "lifestyle choices," are overly simplistic. In his view, individual smokers have lighted their own cigarettes; therefore, if they subsequently need treatment for lung cancer, they should pay their own bills. Yet the tobacco and advertising industries, along with others providing products used in manufacturing cigarettes, and state and federal agencies that subsidize the tobacco industry, have all played significant roles in the chain of events leading up to a smoker's hospitalization for lung cancer. The responsibility of these third parties in smoking and its ill health consequences must be scrutinized in any adequate moral analysis of the problem.

Gauthier argues that occupationally incurred health care costs should be borne by employers. I interpret his brief statements in the following way: not only are employers responsible in the sense of having directed employees to engage in activities that have been harmful to their health, but also employers presumably have benefited from these activities, and could perhaps be said to be the primary beneficiaries. Apparently he sees smokers as responsible for their own health costs not only because they have chosen to smoke, but also because they are the ones who benefit from this activity. But the analogy breaks down. Smokers have not been directed to smoke in the sense that employees have been directed to act in ways that expose them to risk, but smokers do benefit from smoking insofar as they derive pleasure from it. It is not clear, however, that smokers are the primary beneficiaries of smoking. Corporations involved in the promotion and sale of tobacco clearly benefit in a much more straightforward way, a fact that is relevant in considering who should bear the costs of the medical treatment of smokers with lung cancer. Moreover, it is difficult to dispute the contention that the tobacco industry has deliberately exploited

the addictive potential of smoking; given the evidence of the tobacco industry's manipulation of nicotine levels to enhance addictiveness (Schwartz
1994), the assumption that to continue smoking is a fully voluntary, autonomous choice is itself problematic. On the whole, Gauthier's individualistic model of responsibility is inappropriately narrow in this context.[3]

In Gauthier's view, health care needs arise on a generally "accidental" basis, in a context of relatively unimpeded individual choice, and health states
are largely autonomous from other sociopolitical issues. This is an instance
of the "affliction" view of illness as a departure from a world that is otherwise generally orderly and coherent. I take this outlook not only to be inadequate for accommodating the complexities of health, but also to reinforce a defense of an inegalitarian status quo in which corporations
continue to profit to the detriment of individuals, and poor urban communities of color face serious health risks while others benefit.

Daniels's Equality of Opportunity Concept

Daniels is far more attuned than Gauthier to the political and sociocultural
factors affecting health. He provides an expansive categorization of health
care needs, including those goods and services that are necessary

> to maintain, restore, or provide functional equivalents (where possible) to
> normal species functioning. They can be divided into:
>   1 Adequate nutrition, shelter
>   2 Sanitary, safe, unpolluted living and working conditions
>   3 Exercise, rest, and some other features of life-style
>   4 Preventive, curative, and rehabilitative personal medical services
>   5 Non-medical personal and social support services. (1985, 32)

Such a categorization of health care needs is compatible with the recognition that health is socially constituted. Daniels defends health regulations
such as those mandated by the federal Occupational Safety and Health
Administration (OSHA) and provides an interesting account of "quasi-
coerciveness," in which the social context can undercut the autonomy of
choices in consent to occupational risks. This point is worth addressing in

some detail; it provides a useful example of the potential advantages of the distributive paradigm—as well as its limitations (which I take up later in the chapter).

The fair equality of opportunity account mandates an equitable distribution of the risk of disease and injury, insofar as social policy can accomplish this end, and do so in a manner that is compatible with other aspects of justice. This concern for equity motivates Daniels's defense of OSHA-style health regulations in the workplace, in contrast to the view that they interfere unduly with workers' autonomy in consenting to risk. He argues that they do not do so, because the alleged autonomy in this context is largely illusory.

Daniels considers a situation quasi-coercive "if it imposes or depends on a restriction of someone's alternatives in a way that is *unfair* or unjust; that is, a just or fair social arrangement would involve a range of options both broader than and strongly preferred to the range in the proposal situation" (172). The difference between quasi-coercive and "straightforwardly coercive" (171) situations is the indirectness of the former: the "indirect, yet pervasive erosion of that space [the "choice-space" of the individual] as a result of unjust or unfair social practices and institutions. The two share the feature that the restriction is *socially caused*. . . . Moreover, there are just, feasible alternatives" (172).

He argues persuasively that consent to long-term occupational risks such as exposure to chemicals and radiation is just such a situation. First, exposure to most occupational toxins tends to impose invisible and cumulative risks which thus have a "low graspability," unlike the obvious and immediate risks entailed, for example, by firefighting. Also unlike the hazards of firefighting—associated with extraordinary bravery and heroism—long-term exposure to toxins offers no direct intrinsic rewards, just the extrinsic reward of hazard pay. Furthermore, many workers have very few meaningful alternatives to hazardous work. New risks also can emerge when manufacturing processes are changed, and punitive consequences are likely to be imposed for attempting to avoid these risks, such as "possible losses in benefits, pensions, family disruption" (174).

Daniels argues moreover that "it is sufficient that we believe that the restricted range of options such workers enjoy, though fair or just now, would tip in the direction of injustice and unfairness over the long run.

Moreover, we should be concerned that the 'tipping' might be hard to detect and therefore that the quasi-coerciveness would remain hidden and invisible to many participants in the hazard pay market" (175). Thus Daniels defends the imposition of "prior, protective constraints on the framework of markets built on exchanges between workers and employers" (175). This analysis is a useful departure from more simplistic understandings of choice which often result in "blaming the victim," as if individuals were responsible not only for their own decisions but also for the limited range of options they face. Daniels's account is a valuable step toward a more sophisticated analysis of consent, choice, and coercion in the context of an array of social policies and material and historical circumstances which, though not deterministic in the strong sense, nevertheless exert a profound influence on the lives of individuals.

Overall, Daniels's awareness of social inequities in health and health care functions to support his general argument that health care is a good whose distribution requires special care. His fair equality of opportunity account mandates an equitable distribution of the risk of disease and injury, insofar as social policy can accomplish this end, and do so in a manner that is compatible with other aspects of justice; this is a far more careful and considered argument than Gauthier's, and more sensitive to the concerns of at least some of those at risk in the current social context. This account is also inadequate, however, insofar as it deals with specific and unrelated "inequities" rather than the differential treatment, health status, and other concerns of various social groups. In order to lay the groundwork for this argument, a detailed account of Christopher Boorse's empirical notion of health (1987, 1981, 1976) is needed.

Boorse's Descriptive Notion of Health

Christopher Boorse defends an account of health conceptualized strictly in terms of physiological medicine (1981); he argues that even mental health, if there is such a thing, must be conceptualized in analogous terms, which he conceives as "part-functions of the mind" (1987). This empirical notion of health is in contrast to what he sees as a widespread clinical and philosophical consensus "that health is an essentially evaluative notion," and an increasing "tendency . . . to debate social issues in psychiatric terms" (1981, 3).[4] Boorse wants to contest "the recurrent fantasy that what society or its professionals disapprove of is ipso facto unhealthy" (1981, 21). He emphasizes that the notion of health is strictly empirical or descriptive, rather than an evaluative concept or ideal. On his view, "'disease' is simply synonymous with 'unhealthy condition'" (1981, 4), while "illness" is a more specific term referring only to those diseases that exhibit "certain normative features reflected in the institutions of medical practice. An illness must be, first, a reasonably *serious* disease with incapacitating effects which make it undesirable. . . . Secondly, to call a disease an illness is to view its owner as deserving special treatment and diminished moral accountability" (1981, 10). The concept of illness, then, is similar to the sociological concept of the "sick role," a normative judgment (Daniels 1985, 29) whose application varies with the norms of particular societies, whereas attributions of disease are not relative to specific settings. Boorse seems to abandon this distinction in his later work (1987), yet nonetheless retains the empirical, nonrelativist concept of disease as unhealthy condition.

The physiological concept of health turns on the notion of species-typical function: "Diseases . . . interfere with one or more functions typically performed within members of the species" (1981, 12), and the central goals this model identifies for any species are survival and reproduction. Boorse argues that the concept of health is thus "strictly analogous to the mechanical condition of an artifact . . . the conformity of the process to a fixed design" (1981, 13). Design in the case of organisms refers to statistical normality. His later work refines this definition further: "Health is *normal functioning*, and what is pathological is *abnormal* functioning. . . . A condition of a part or process in an organism is *pathological* when the ability of the part or process to perform one or more of its species-typical biological functions falls below some central range of the statistical distribution for that ability in corresponding parts or processes in members of an appropriate reference class of the species" (1987, 370).

Boorse notes that this view provides a fairly clear-cut distinction between "core" and "peripheral" medicine: medicine in the core sense involves "the removal, mitigation, or prevention of pathology. . . . The justification for medical therapy in the core sense is that normal biological functional ability is almost always desirable" (1987, 383–84). Medical treatments that do not meet this definition (such as cosmetic surgery, for example) therefore fall into the realm of peripheral medicine, which Boorse does not oppose but believes that "it usually lacks the objectivity and moral urgency of the medicine of health promotion" (383). This distinction supports the related distinction in the literature between health care "needs" and health care "demands" (which may or may not constitute needs). In both distinctions, necessary uses of health care are conceptualized in terms of biomedical theory.

On the face of it, it may seem that this account may exclude some universal or near-universal conditions in a particular society which are generally understood to be diseases, such as ubiquitous tooth decay (1981, 13). Boorse notes, however, that such conditions are still "deviation[s] from the natural functional organization of the species" (13) and are generally environmentally caused. Thus, "deficiencies in the functional efficiency of the body are diseases when they are unnatural, and they may be unnatural either by being atypical or by being attributable mainly to the action of a hostile environment" (13).

Daniels subscribes to this descriptive notion of health and disease, using the concept of health as normal species functioning to ground a characterization of health care needs, which he argues must be both "objectively ascribable" and "objectively important," that is, carrying significant moral weight (1985, 25). For Daniels, this account draws "a fairly sharp line between uses of health-care services to prevent and treat diseases and uses which meet other social goals" (31). Gauthier endorses this notion as well (1983); both he and Daniels explicitly reject the World Health Organization's definition of health as "a state of complete physical, mental, and social well-being, and not merely the absence of disease or infirmity" (cited in Daniels 1985, 29). Daniels argues, "Health is not happiness, and confusing the two over-medicalizes social philosophy" (29). Thus, Gauthier and Daniels concur that the descriptive account provides a useful way of avoiding this confusion.

But this account, meant to eliminate the controversies associated with evaluative theories of health and to avoid certain problems of social relativism, fails on both counts. It indeed represents a vital recognition that characterizations of specific diseases are sometimes based on social disapproval of a given condition, which does not render it pathological by any means; many such characterizations are largely based on hidden and therefore undefended social values. For example, Boorse notes "the tendency to call radical activists, bohemians, feminists, and other unpopular deviants [including "homosexuals"] 'sick'" (1981, 21–22), referring not only to popular usage but to psychiatry as well. Nevertheless, several elements of the descriptive health account implicitly rely on undefended evaluative assumptions that function to reinforce traditional social values—a serious charge given that this account is meant to avoid morally and politically evaluative notions altogether.

First of all, the descriptive account ostensibly excludes subjective factors from the criteria for health and disease. The supposedly jointly sufficient conditions of the atypicality or environmental genesis of a physical state and its deviation from an organism's functional "design," deny any definitional significance to the subjective states of pain and suffering. Edmund Pellegrino describes illness as an experience of "ontological rupture," a state of existential vulnerability in which one's "freedom to act as a person is severely compromised" (1982, 159). Pellegrino argues, "Genuine healing must be based on an authentic perception of the experience of illness in *this* person" (160). In the previous chapter I argued against an ontological understanding of illness in abstraction from the social context. Pellegrino's account, however, is useful in illuminating the significance of subjectivity, which I see as crucial to the conceptualization of illness. For example, in the medicalization of menstruation, discussed in Chapter 1, women may receive medical treatment despite a lack of subjective suffering (or because of others' suffering rather than their own), while others may not receive the treatment they seek, or their subjective complaints may be minimized, as has often been the case with menstrual pain. The subjective experiences of members of oppressed groups are an important social resource in the struggle to overcome injustice, a claim that is significant for the understanding of both health and disease. One of the reasons why homosexuality was abandoned as a psychiatric diagnosis was that members of the profession finally listened to the claim that being gay did not inherently entail psychological suffering.

A further problem with Boorse's account is that conceptualizing human health in terms of the "species-goals" of survival and reproduction confuses individual states or needs with those of a species, employing an abstract classificatory concept to describe the states of individuals.[5] Although species survival is clearly a necessary condition for the mere existence, and perhaps even the well-being, of any of its members, it certainly is not a sufficient condition for individual health. Furthermore, whereas a *species* must produce offspring in order to survive, reproduction is not necessary for a particular individual's health or survival.[6]

The fundamental problem here is that defining health in reproductive terms involves a teleological interpretation of human biology (Martin 1987) with profoundly moral and political implications. In some cases Boorse seems unaware of these influences of traditional morality in medical discourse, while in other cases he accepts them. In his attempt "to analyze the normal-pathological distinction in traditional medicine," Boorse notes, "a correct analysis, or reportive definition, must conform to medical usage—that is, it must fit the stock of recognized pathological conditions. Definitions that are wider or narrower than [this] stock are incorrect. For example, traditional medicine never describes pregnancy, menstruation, male or female fertility, penile foreskins, or Oriental ancestry as pathological, or as diseases" (1987, 366). Yet, as I illustrated in Chapter 1, traditional medicine does pathologize the menstrual cycle both subtly and overtly, and despite its teleological understanding of female biology in reproductive terms, it nonetheless also pathologizes pregnancy and childbirth by treating them as one long emergency requiring medical intervention.

In addition, as I argued in Chapter 2, it is this same teleology that also pathologizes gay male and lesbian sexuality, thereby building a sexist and heterosexist bias into theories of health. On this view, all women, whether heterosexual or not, are defined reproductively, as mothers (potential, actual, or failed); and gay and bisexual men are perceived as biological aberrations. Boorse (who refers repeatedly to homosexuality as a "perversion," a word with clear moral overtones, its status as a psychological term notwithstanding) is quite clear on the latter point: "On general biological principles, the exclusive homosexual (but not the bisexual) looks pathological by virtue of his or her reproductive failure. Some recent biologists suggest models (e.g., kin selection) by which evolution could favor genes for homosexuality in the population. Unless some such model is vindicated, exclusive homosexuality seems likely to be a form of mental pathology, as psychoanalysts have always maintained" (1987, 385).

It is difficult to know what to make of this view. On the one hand, Boorse notes that "homosexuality . . . might be a minor form of pathology, like a wart or red-green color blindness, and one as consistent with happiness as any other abnormality . . . producing infertility" (1987, 385). Yet he also states that "if homosexuality were shown both pathological and contagious to young children, that might justify disqualifying homosexuals from teaching elementary school" (386), evoking the absurd yet pernicious notion of moral contagion which occurs so frequently in this issue.

As I have illustrated in the context of gynecology and obstetrics, heterosexuality becomes an implicit medical and moral norm, while human biology is defined in terms of (heterosexual) maleness. In many contexts (as I will argue subsequently), biomedical discourse defines heterosexual men primarily as healthy adults and only secondarily as fathers, despite the overall reproductive bias. This implicit male norm is in contrast to femaleness, which is defined in terms of two states: the special case of pregnancy, which is pathologized in certain ways, versus the special and (differently) pathologized states of non-pregnant femaleness. Ruth Hubbard notes that "the most fundamental theory in biology—the theory of evolution by natural selection—is constructed around sex and procreation" (1990, 139). She attributes this conceptual structure to the historical influence of sexual dichotomy as a central feature of the social context.

The framing of species design in reproductive terms can be understood as the expression of social norms. Emily Martin points out, for example, that the nineteenth century brought increasing emphasis on a sexual dimorphism which was both descriptive and prescriptive, defining women (especially upper- and middle-class white women) as mothers, and relegating them to the home in accord with the doctrine of separate spheres (1987, 31–33).[7] Not coincidentally, at this time, in contrast to earlier views, menstruation came increasingly to be defined as a disorder, thereby pathologizing femaleness itself (34–35). Other critics have identified ways in which evolutionary theory has translated historical conditions under industrialized capitalism (such as a hierarchical social structure) into universal "facts of nature" (Janson-Smith, 1980).

Moreover, the attribution of a "fixed design" to the human species is another means of positing the clear and distinct boundary between the natural and the social which I argue must be resisted. This sharp dichotomy

ignores the inseparability of biology from human action and social practice, which should be central to any understanding of human physiology
and health-related needs.[8] Historically this idea has functioned to support
traditional views of social roles, and thus requires moral evaluation. Ruth
Hubbard views science in the nineteenth century as functioning conser-
vatively "to replace the waning ideological power of the church by bol-
stering or replacing God's laws with laws of nature" (1990, 36). She rejects
"biodeterminist" theories of human nature or fixed essence, advocating instead a dialectic, contextualized understanding of human physiology, existing transformationally "in dynamic interaction with our environment"
(138), which includes politics and social arrangements. I see her critique of
nineteenth-century science as a vital reminder to continue to interrogate
the cultural mythology encoded in medicine, an aspect of the discourse
which Boorse seems to assume has perished in the dawn of more recent scientific progress.

Despite Boorse's sharp criticism of science's infiltration by the values of
those who would define mental health, for example, in terms of the qualities they themselves esteem or the traits favored by society, there are certainly social influences at work in his own views. Sometimes he openly es-
pouses certain values, such as his disapproval of feminist psychotherapy on
the grounds that it is similar to "Soviet psychiatrists diagnosing political dis-
sidence as 'sluggish schizophrenia': in both cases, the vocabulary of medicine is being used to mask political ends" (1987, 384). Never mind that one
case involves the use of state power to silence dissidents, while the other,
based on the claims of the feminist therapist Boorse cites, involves training
women to become assertive, overcome inhibitions, and recognize personal
rights—surely very different uses of therapeutic discourse. This example
of Boorse's indicates what I see as a fundamental failure of his analysis: its
inability to address power relationships in the context of medicine.

At other times the values that influence his perspectives are less overt, as
in his theory of mental health (1987). He argues that a concept of mental
health should be modeled after the empirical physiological view of health,
not as a physiological conception, but rather by providing an account of
parts and functions of the mind. He believes that psychoanalytic theory offers such an account; moreover, despite the problem of cultural variation
in standards of psychological normality, he believes nonetheless that "it

may be possible to state universal criteria of normality at a deeper level of psychological theory" (378). On his view, such criteria "might include freedom from crippling anxiety, deep and stable love relations, full and unconflicted development of one's abilities, and the capacity for orgasmic sexual release" (378).

It is not clear to me how these criteria are purely descriptive rather than the expression of an ideal. More important, even though these traits might well be desirable in any society, and thus not merely the expression of Boorse's personal values or the values of this particular society, it is important to understand how attributions of these traits function in the present context. Although these traits may be objectively desirable in some sense, they clearly are not universally valued as a measure that applies to everyone alike. In contemporary U.S. society, moreover, they may well disproportionately describe (or perhaps be attributed to) the privileged. As a group, women have had far fewer opportunities than men for the "full and unconflicted development" of our abilities, and have been encouraged to put aside personal goals and aspirations for the sake of families.

Members of other oppressed groups have been denied opportunities as well. In fact, a social environment that fosters domestic violence, rape, and anti-gay hate crimes is likely to impose difficulties in each of Boorse's four areas, which are not rooted in individual psychopathology, while the batterer, the rapist, or the gay-basher may even seem healthier than the survivor on at least some of these criteria.

Perhaps Boorse would respond that it is only right, after all, to identify any absence of these traits as unideal, since it is in everyone's interests to possess them. He might also add that the theory addresses environmental causation, in that certain conditions that may be widespread or even typical may nonetheless be diseases if environmentally caused. Such a response is not adequate, however, because this analysis fails to address the harmful conditions that are socially created, stopping short by locating the problem in the individual rather than in power imbalances structured into social relations. Given that the chief value of concepts of health and disease is their use in diagnosing and treating problems, without an analysis of the social context in which psychological traits arise and have meaning, Boorse's proposed mental health criteria may create more problems than they solve.

One may find these criticisms persuasive yet still ask whether this empirical account of health may yet be salvaged. Some of Boorse's comments, particularly those on mental health, may not necessarily reflect on the core aspects of the empirical account. I explore this question next in the context of Gauthier's and Daniels's understanding of specific women's health concerns.

Issues in Women's Health

When Daniels discusses health issues related to women, reproduction is usually involved in some way—which is not the case in reference to men (or to gender-neutral "persons" or "workers"). Although associating women but not men with reproduction might seem to be an attempt to address the specificity of women's experiences and the health care needs they generate, this practice actually serves to reinforce the social ideology of female selflessness, of women as beings-for-others, and to exacerbate other disadvantages to women, imposing special costs on them in a variety of ways. This can be seen in the context of Daniels's views on certain occupational health measures related to childbearing as well as other women's health issues, which not only are socially occasioned in ways that Gauthier and Daniels do not recognize, but also are strongly related to the broader issue of women's autonomy and personal agency.

Daniels discusses women's health concerns only in relation to childbearing: prenatal and maternal/infant care, or the "special sensitivity" of pregnant women to occupational hazards such as airborne lead. Implicitly, women but not men are defined reproductively. Daniels fails to address some very problematic aspects of "special sensitivity" and "fetal vulnerability" policies, despite his concern to protect the opportunities of the most "sensitive." The ways in which sensitivity is defined, by whom, and with subsequent benefit for whom, and the context of labor practices in which such definitions are applied, go unexamined. For example, directing protective policies only toward women, and only on the basis of potential fetal harm, is itself problematic. The effects of lead exposure also include damage to sperm—although men are not defined as being at risk reproductively—as well as risks to the health of both male and female workers themselves. (Thus, the very term "special sensitivity" is a misnomer.) Yet not only are women's opportunities restricted in this context in an inappropriately differential manner, but also the full range of hazards is not addressed. While some male workers may gain economic opportunities at the expense of some female workers, the hazards remain, and corporations may benefit at the expense of workers and their families.

In some cases women have been required to offer proof of sterilization or else lose their jobs. Strikingly, such "protection" occurs most often in occupations traditionally held by men; the hazards faced by women in traditionally female jobs are much less likely to be regulated (Hubbard 1990, 26). Deirdre Janson-Smith writes of the power of sociobiological definitions of women in reproductive terms, arguing that the prominence of such views is determined by "the varying need for female labour" (1980, 86). And Ruth Hubbard argues that biological theories of sex difference (particularly in terms of reproductive functions) work "to rationalize the stratification of the labor force by sex" (1990, 124). In short, it is important to evaluate critically the overall social context from which such policies emerge, and to consider their impact on society as a whole as well as on specific groups. These policies do not occur in a vacuum, nor do they occur in a context that recognizes women's rights as workers. Rather, they are part of a labor context in which discrimination against women, and failure to respect the interests of workers in general, takes many forms.

Daniels tends to overlook the interests of women *themselves*, apart from their capacity as actual or potential mothers. The vulnerability of fetuses functions differentially to constrain women's but not men's choices, while other health risks to women, men, and children are overlooked, so that women in these occupations who will become mothers cannot earn the same wages as men who may or may not become fathers. At the same time, the descriptive account defines as actual and legitimate only those health needs associated with pregnancy and childbirth, not with their prevention. Thus certain social practices are recast as facts of nature, with some side effects that happen to affect women in unfortunate ways. Women's "special sensitivity" owing to the "vulnerability" of actual or potential fetuses is an instance of the conflict between women's roles as mothers and as wage earners, which is rooted not so much in women's bodies as in the social relations that structure women's lives.

A host of environmental toxins is known to cause complications in pregnancy and fetal development, and these toxins come in such a variety of forms that it is generally difficult for pregnant women to avoid exposure to at least some of them (Norwood 1985). Yet efforts are directed toward excluding women of childbearing age from certain jobs in which exposure is likely, and blaming individual women or restricting their behavior in other ways, rather than toward eradicating these toxins to the fullest extent possible. Joan Bertin of the American Civil Liberties Union comments, "If you have a health and safety problem, you fix the workplace, not the worker. If something made your spleen become infected at work, you wouldn't say, 'We'll only take workers who don't have spleens'" (Cohen 1990). Identifying these socially occasioned risks to health as exceptional overlooks systematic labor practices that treat the health of individuals as expendable (or compensable, as in Gauthier's view).

I turn now to several significant women's health issues which are intimately connected to the social context, and which Gauthier and Daniels either do not address or treat inadequately.

Domestic Violence

Domestic violence, first of all, "is the single most frequent cause of injury to women—more frequent than mugging, rape, and auto accidents combined. Half of all American women are assaulted by their husbands or male companions at least once" (Erlanger 1989, 81). Each year male partners assault at least 2 million women—a figure some researchers believe may be half the actual number because of underreporting (Colburn 1994). Four thousand women are murdered in the United States each year by their partners (Erlanger 1989, 81), and the American Medical Association attributes 25 percent of female suicides to domestic violence (Colburn 1994). Violence apparently begins early: 25 percent of teenage girls in the United States report that they have experienced physical violence from boyfriends (Shen 1993). Magazine articles and television movies lament domestic violence in the tragic language used for natural disasters and acts of God; yet, as Richard Gelles and Murray Straus note, "the amount of money allocated to prevent and treat private violence and abuse is so small that it would be considered a rounding error in the Defense Department" (1988, 187)—a statement that neatly clarifies the nation's social priorities.

Such a widespread phenomenon as domestic violence cannot be dismissed as the isolated actions of a few pathologically disturbed individuals. Instead, the problem must be understood as an expression of patriarchal power relations, an interpretation supported by a growing body of research. Based on their analysis of 34,000 police reports, 933 police and court cases, and interviews with 109 female survivors, R. Emerson and Russell Dobash recognize family violence as an expression of social ideals of marriage and gender relations, functioning "as the extension of the domination and control of husbands over wives. . . . Violence in the family should be understood primarily as coercive control" (1979, 15). Such violence is not simply the result of a spontaneous outburst of temper, loss of control, or personal or familial dysfunction; it is a practice by which men gain power over women.

Moreover, the control practiced by individual men is supported by patriarchal social structure and ideology (Dobash and Dobash 1979, 43–44), and by institutions that respond inappropriately, offer rationales or justifications for the violence, discourage women from leaving or resisting, or fail to intervene or to support women adequately.[9] In many cases male batterers' patriarchal control of women may also be supported or tolerated by other men around them. A frequent theme in the research literature is the number of ways in which batterers' male friends condone their behavior. Lee H. Bowker's study of one thousand domestic violence survivors attributes domestic violence to "the masculine culture of violence" (1986, 103). He found that batterers' male friends often reinforce the acceptability of violence (102–4, 113): "The more frequently a man socialized with his friends, the more severely and extensively he battered his wife" (102). According to Dobash and Dobash, "The woman's friends or relations are much more likely to intervene than the husband's" (1979, 113).

Many researchers convincingly argue that gender relations must be transformed in order to solve the problem. Bowker concludes that only "a shift in the marital power balance" will stop domestic violence (1986, 98). Similarly, Gelles and Straus call for "the elimination of sexism" as a necessary condition for remedying the problem. They also call for mandatory reporting by police and physicians, as well as mandatory arrest; perinatal screening by doctors; [10] intervention and support services; and universal access to health care, including family planning and abortion services, as necessary aspects of women's empowerment (1988, 191–206).

In summary, the harm that men inflict on women in domestic violence is socially supported and reinforced to a significant degree. It must be understood that women face a high risk of domestic violence, and that this phenomenon exemplifies the power relations at work in the creation and constitution of health care needs. Domestic violence is not an affliction that happens to befall some women randomly but a clear expression of social relations and values. This problem cannot adequately be addressed within the constraints of the distributive paradigm of justice. Expanding access to health care is not a sufficient response; preventing and treating the problem requires social transformation.

Obstetric and Gynecological Surgeries

Beyond domestic violence, the distributive paradigm offers no account of how the institution of medicine is implicated in other problems such as creating unnecessary health care "needs." The women's health movement has produced an extensive body of literature on illness and injury directly caused by gynecology and obstetrics. [11] The practice of medicine itself gives rise to specific health care uses in two ways: through iatrogenesis (disease or injury caused by the practice of medicine) and through the medical creation of demands (such as the recommendation of unnecessary or overly extensive services).

The high rate of gynecological surgery is a case in point. Many sterilizations, radical mastectomies, cesarean sections, and hysterectomies are performed unnecessarily, or when less intrusive and equally legitimate forms of treatment are available (Ruzek 1978, 49–52). The Hysterectomy Education Resources and Services group "has counseled more than 13,000 women who were told they needed hysterectomies, and referred them to other physicians for second opinions . . . [and] 98 percent of those women were told by other doctors they did not need the surgery" (Baron-Faust 1989, 193). In a study of seven health maintenance organizations, 16 percent of 642 hysterectomies performed were found to be "clearly unnecessary," and another 25 percent "were of questionable value" ("HMO Study" 1993). Cesarean sections are also frequently performed without necessity—500,000 yearly, according to the Public Citizen Health Research Group ("Study Supports Suspicions" 1993), which estimated that eliminating unnecessary C-sections "could save about $1.3 billion in medical costs" (Brown 1994). The physical, emotional, and economic consequences of these major surgeries must not be underestimated.

The rise in these health care uses reflects more than the economic interests of doctors. It is related on a deeper level to the modern medical paradigm, with its uncritical faith in technological intervention and in medical authority itself as the means of solving human problems. In gynecology and obstetrics, patriarchal mistrust of women's bodies is added to these core beliefs (Daly 1978). Sue Fisher identifies "certain crucial beliefs about women and the delivery of health care . . . [which] are displayed and maintained in gynecological textbooks, in articles in medical journals, and perhaps most importantly, in day-to-day medical practices." For example, "many doctors believe that once a woman is through reproducing, she no longer needs her uterus . . . [and] that the prophylactic removal of a uterus not only sterilizes a woman, but also reduces the likelihood that her uterus will become diseased. . . . They believe that the birth control pill is safer than unwanted pregnancy . . . [and] that they are the appropriate ones to be making medical decisions" (1986, 6–7). While it may seem self-evident to some that doctors are the proper authorities on "medical decisions," what must be remembered is that these decisions cannot be separated from the context of individual women's lives: these are life decisions, moral questions, as much as they are "medical" ones. Thus, the distributive paradigm's inattention to the authority ceded to medicine represents a failure to examine not only an important aspect of health care but the deeper problem of the social control of women's lives as well.

This medical authority over women, moreover, is only intensified for women of color and poor women, who in the United States and Puerto Rico have faced sterilization abuse in the guise of population control. Angela Davis notes the large number of women sterilized in 1972 alone: "Carl Schultz, director of [the Department of Health, Education and Welfare's] Population Affairs Office, estimated that between 100,000 and

200,000 sterilizations had actually been funded that year by the federal government" (1981, 218). She compares this figure to the "250,000 sterilizations . . . carried out under the Nazis' Hereditary Health Law" (218). By the 1970s, 24 percent of Native American women in the reproductive years, and 20 percent of Latinas as well as married African American women, had been sterilized (218–19). Many hysterectomies, known to southern black women as "Mississippi appendectomies," were performed without the patient's consent, particularly in the 1960s and 1970s (Ruzek 1978, 46–47). Numerous women of color and poor white women have been sterilized coercively or under less than fully informed and voluntary conditions (Corea 1985, Dreifus 1977, Poirier 1990).

More recently, Native American women have criticized the Indian Health Service's administration of the contraceptive implant Norplant. Among this group are high rates of various risk factors for the drug, yet in many regions the Indian Health Service actively promotes it, frequently without adequate counseling about risks and side effects—despite a 1987 federal investigation into IHS mishandling of Depo Provera, another contraceptive drug (Native American Women 1993, 69). In all these cases, policy makers' goal of controlling the growth of populations of color dovetails with the gynecological control of women's lives, resulting in infringements of women's rights.

Far from being "afflictions" that happen to befall some women, these obstetrical and gynecological problems exemplify the ways in which specific social practices and ideologies not only create unnecessary health care uses for women but also violate women's bodily integrity. The distributive paradigm neither addresses this problem nor recognizes how gynecology perpetuates a view of the female body as inherently problematic, requiring medical mediation and intervention. Like domestic violence, this too is an external interference with women's physical and mental health which is supported by patriarchal social relations.

Abortion

Abortion is also embedded in a context of social practices and ideologies which are insufficiently addressed by theorists such as Daniels and Gauthier.

The descriptive account of health grounding their theories excludes "nontherapeutic" abortion and contraception from the realm of health care needs. Since on this account health is understood as "the absence of disease," seen as "deviations from the natural functional organization of a typical member of a species," health care is conceived as "care aimed at preventing or reducing deviations in natural functional organization" (1983, 180). Gauthier can only conclude from this that "providing health care" does not involve "providing abortions for those whose normal functioning is not impaired by pregnancy (which itself must be understood as a natural human condition)" (205). For Boorse, abortion is a peripheral rather than a core use of medicine, "because a fetus is not pathology[,] and unhappiness [resulting from unwanted pregnancy] is not ill health" (1987, 383). Daniels also concurs that abortion is not a health care need (he sees this as a "minor implication" of the descriptive account of health), although he does leave open the possibility that there may be other reasons for public funding of at least some abortions (1985, 31–32). Gauthier objects not to the availability of abortions for those who can pay for them, but rather to the use of public funds to help allay the cost of some abortions on the basis of financial need. While neither Daniels nor Gauthier discusses contraception,[12] Boorse identifies it, like abortion, as a peripheral use of medicine. Moreover, in theories of access to health care based on the descriptive account of health, it seems clear that contraception is not a health care need, at least for those women whose health would not be seriously jeopardized by pregnancy and birth: if pregnancy is not a deviation from species-typical function, then neither is its prevention a case of treating or preventing disease.

Far from its being a "minor implication" of the descriptive account, excluding abortion and contraception reveals deep conceptual problems. This framework excludes an important demand for many women, ignores the social constitution of sexuality and its role in our lives, minimizes the profound effects of a woman's ability to control pregnancy upon her life prospects, and creates an artificial boundary between "health care needs" and other services which "happen" to be provided in that context.

According to the Alan Guttmacher Institute, "46 percent of American women have abortions at some point in their lives, often because of contraceptive failure, which accounts for 30 million pregnancies a year round the world" (Mann 1994). No contraceptive is entirely effective, and "birth control failure is highest among poor, unmarried and minority women" ("New Study" 1989), for whom an unwanted pregnancy is likely to create disproportionate burdens.

On Gauthier's view, pregnancy might well epitomize a personal lifestyle choice, resulting as it does from an act of intercourse by an individual woman and man. Yet this "individual" act does not occur apart from the social world; in fact, the heterosexual nature of this intercourse is itself socially mandated. Adrienne Rich has written persuasively of our society's "compulsory heterosexuality" (1980). Society enforces this mandate by various means, such as social stigma, familial pressure or rejection, the refusal to grant gay and lesbian couples the social status and other rights and benefits of heterosexual marriage, barriers to child custody, discrimination in employment and in the enforcement of sodomy laws, and widespread hostility and violence against those who are lesbian or gay, or are perceived to be so.[13] As long as lesbianism is discouraged in these and other ways while heterosexuality and marriage continue to be promoted, it will be impossible to distinguish in any meaningful way between "natural" versus socially created needs for contraception, abortion, and reproductive care.

It is important to acknowledge that what is at stake in the abortion issue is the ability to make choices not merely about "family planning" but about sexuality as well. We are bombarded daily with sexualized images in the mass media, yet the ability to make personal sexual choices is seldom treated as a right worth defending—especially for women, for whom dealing with sexual intimidation and coercion is a standard part of our socialization. Few defend the rights of mothers on public assistance, for example, to make sexual choices other than celibacy. Sexual choice is indeed a highly significant element in the pursuit of the good life, expressing an individual's values and desires in a uniquely intimate way; interference with these choices is thus uniquely intrusive as well. While few would go so far as to advocate policing the sexual behavior of women receiving public assistance, access to a full range of choices is commonly regarded as an economic privilege which must be earned. Feminists correctly identify access to abortion and contraception not only as a key measure of women's health but also as a necessary safeguard for such choices.

Because neither Gauthier nor Daniels addresses the role of sexuality in life choices, both overlook the impact of social practices related to sexuality on the status of women as a group, their life prospects, and opportunities.[14] When women have no way to end or avoid an unwanted pregnancy, a special cost is imposed on them, not just for their own sexual choices but for those of their male sexual partners as well. Thus charges of injustice may be leveled not only against legal barriers to abortion and contraception, but also against the failure to guarantee that all women, regardless of socioeconomic standing, have access to these safeguards. Otherwise, only the sexual self-determination of (heterosexual) men is preserved, while women who can afford contraceptive and reproductive care are taking on a special cost, and women who cannot afford such care take on a much greater burden. Such discrepancies create distinct social advantages for heterosexual men, as well as for some heterosexually active women over others.

These theorists' treatment of abortion has important consequences for both social constraints on sexual choices and life prospects in general. Gauthier's position on public funding of abortion as a health care need (and by implication contraception as well) is connected to a libertarian view of justice. A central aspect of this ideal is noninterference with individuals' pursuit of the good life as they conceive it, to the extent that that is compatible with an equivalent degree of noninterference for all, and with other social goals. In Gauthier's view, any theory of fairness in access to health care must be compatible with this overarching goal of noninterference (as distinct from a more liberal view of positive entitlements).

As for Daniels, whose general outlook is of the Rawlsian liberal persuasion rather than the libertarian, it is perhaps more surprising (especially given Daniels's focus on opportunity) that he makes no connection between access to abortion and the general life prospects of women and of their partners and families as well. There are not only economic concerns here, but also issues of control over one's body (a concern that Daniels mentions [32]), as well as the traditional liberal value of control over one's life — the pursuit of the good life as one conceives it. This good is clearly less available to women than to men if access to abortion is not secured.

Women disproportionately bear the day-to-day responsibilities of child care, and thus a woman's ability to choose whether or not to bear and raise a child influences her life prospects — indeed, her very ability to control her life—to a degree that few other discrete choices do. Given the disproportionate nature of this responsibility, providing contraception and abortion is one tool (along with adequate support for other options) for undermining existing social inequities between women and men. Since President Clinton's notorious difficulty in nominating a candidate for attorney general, there has been more awareness than ever of the scarcity of child care arrangements that serve the needs of parents and children while complying with tax codes and immigration law—and affordability is of course a much greater problem for the vast majority of the population, who are not as financially privileged as Clinton's attorney general candidates. Once again, a gender differential is at work: it is female parents whose employment status and job security are most likely to be at risk after the birth of a child.

Since the public sector is not structured around the needs of children and their caretakers (Wendell 1989), mothers who work outside the home must often interrupt their employment for long periods, or reduce their aspirations, resulting in the loss of income just when needs are greatest. Some women deal with child care needs by taking up home-based employment, which often lacks adequate benefits. Women used to paid employment outside the home may also suffer isolation and a loss of self-esteem when they stay at home. Mothers whose partners are employed risk economic dependency on them, while single mothers and those whose partners are not fully employed are at special risk for poverty. Depending on their socioeconomic positions, mothers face varying degrees of material deprivation, yet all but the most affluent risk erosion of autonomy and control over their own life decisions. In addition, when a woman must continue an unplanned pregnancy against her will, profound physical and psychological burdens are imposed which are all the more dramatic given the relative simplicity of the alternative of abortion for those who choose it. Again, all of these consequences accrue to women in ways that are not the case for men, and thus enter into the special costs imposed on women for their male partners' sexual choices in addition to their own.

Many who oppose abortion see adoption as the solution for women facing unplanned pregnancies. This may well be a viable option for some. Yet for others it is not; giving up a baby can be deeply painful and injure a woman's sense of self. Twenty-five years after relinquishing the son born to her at nineteen, Carol Schaefer wrote of this experience: "Mothers who give up their babies inevitably and profoundly alter the rest of their lives. Many cannot go on to lead fulfilling existences, haunted by fear for their child's welfare, guilt both for abandoning their child and for continuing to love and long for him, and shame, too, at having taken the 'easy' way out" (1991, 293–94). Adoptive parents may also face special challenges with little or no acknowledgment, preparation, or support, while many adoptees struggle their whole lives with feelings of isolation, insecurity, and disconnection (Lifton 1979). Although not every birth parent, adoptee, or adoptive parent necessarily experiences these difficulties, they certainly undercut an unreflective faith in adoption as a benign institution in everyone's best interests (Raymond 1994).

All of these decisions—whether to bear children, and if so, when, how many, and under what conditions; whether to continue a pregnancy; whether to raise a child—are among the most significant of human choices, expressing one's desires, values, and commitments, and profoundly influencing the life prospects of a woman and those close to her. Abortion and contraception must be available to all women in order for these choices to be meaningful, and to avoid special costs to women for their sexual choices. Gauthier and Daniels might respond that excluding abortion from the realm of health care needs does not constitute *direct* interference with life prospects. Perhaps they would also claim that in the absence of formal legal barriers to contraception and abortion, individual choice has been preserved in the form of noninterference.

Excluding these needs from the realm of health care, however, overlooks the fact that access to them is an important safeguard for the health of women and children (Lantos 1994). When women—especially poor women—cannot control the number and spacing of births, they and their children face risks to their health. These theorists also overlook the injuries, fatalities, and psychological suffering caused when women attempt to terminate pregnancies without access to safe abortions. Furthermore, a noninterference view of abortion does not address the circumstances of access. Even women who can afford abortion do not necessarily have access to it. A woman may have access to gynecological care and still not have access to abortion: "In 82% of the counties in the U.S., there are no abortion providers" ("Facts" 1990). Gena Corea notes: "In 1979 and 1980, the vast majority of abortions were performed in metropolitan areas. Only

4.5% took place in nonmetropolitan areas, although about 26% of women of reproductive age live in these areas" (1985, 207). The training of providers is also an important factor in access. According to a 1991 study, "only 12 percent of American medical schools and residency programs teach doctors to perform abortions," a drop from 22 percent in 1986 (Boodman 1993). A 1995 survey found that only "one-third of practicing obstetrician-gynecologists perform abortion, a drop from 42 percent in 1983" (Russell 1995, A3). Significantly fewer young obstetrician-gyne-cologists perform abortions than older doctors of the same specialization, "with those over 65 more than twice as likely to do so as their colleagues under 40," according to the same survey. The recent escalation of violence against abortion providers is likely to diminish availability even further.

Ultimately, the very claim that abortion is not a health care need be-cause it is not a treatment for restoring or maintaining species-typical functioning (or compensating for a lack of it) has consequences that many will find objectionable. If pregnancy is not a disease, and a fetus is not a pathology, then the medicalization of normal pregnancy and childbirth (i.e., those not classified as high risk or emergency, leaving aside the issue of the increase in such designations) is no more a "core" use of medicine in Christopher Boorse's sense than abortion (1981). Proponents of the de-scriptive account might respond that childbirth ought to be medicalized because of the risk of potentially serious complications. Yet surely this as-pect of childbirth does not distinguish it from abortion, which—al-though a much simpler process than childbirth—can be risky if per-formed without skill or in unsanitary conditions. A way in which the two are clearly not analogous, however, is that one is socially lauded as the true meaning of womanhood, while the other is deeply controversial, per-ceived as giving women a power that many are reluctant to grant. Thus, in rejecting the status of abortion as a health care need on the grounds of an empirical, ostensibly value-free account of health, these theorists re-produce the undefended social value of pro-natalism.

Contextualizing Sexuality and Health

These health concerns of women are so closely interwoven with the social context as to be socially occasioned to a significant degree. Each has important implications for the personal autonomy of women. In domestic violence, battering functions directly to undermine a woman's autonomy and to diminish her self-esteem and efficacy. In obstetrics and gynecology, unnecessary and sometimes coercive surgery and reproductive control treat women as objects, particularly women of color, compounding the harms of racism which they are already likely to face. Abortion must be understood in the context of powerful social norms: of heterosexuality, and of contraception as a female responsibility, manifested in assumptions about sex education, individual practices in sexual relationships, and medical contraceptive research focused almost exclusively on women. Abortion is an important aspect of women's struggle for both sexual and reproductive autonomy, and is strongly tied to other life choices as well.

On the descriptive account, these concerns are perceived as individual medical needs which are in some sense accidental (ill-fated afflictions), or in the case of abortion, not a medical need at all but a use of medical technology for non-health-related individual purposes. Yet in failing to recognize and challenge women's pervasive disadvantages in relation to men, the descriptive account takes them for granted: batterers benefit at women's expense as marriage is constructed as a relationship of coercive control; physicians (predominantly male), hospitals, and other agencies benefit at the expense of female patients; and heterosexual men benefit at the expense of women. These disadvantages, and the overall erosion of women's autonomy, are all the more striking when one considers that together these health issues constitute a significant share of women's total health care uses—indeed, of overall health care needs in society.

Women's experiences with sexual and reproductive health demonstrate the embeddedness of health problems and needs in the social context. Theorists who do not recognize this are not merely mislocating the boundary between needs that are socially created and those that are not; the very assumption of such a clear-cut geography must be challenged because of the constant interactions between social relations and the physical aspects of human existence. Defining health in terms of "natural and normal human functioning" (Gauthier 1983, 184) simply begs the question if, as I have argued, for human physiology there is no autonomous "natural" existing separately from the social. Measurements of the "normal," moreover, are always mediated through cultural values, and thus must be critically interrogated.

Ultimately Daniels's work has little advantage over Gauthier's in matters of sexuality and health.[15] The problem is not simply that neither theorist addresses matters of sexuality, leaving unchallenged the medical power to define and thereby regulate sexuality; nor is it only the inadvertent privileging of the interests of male heterosexuals over others which occurs when women are defined in reproductive terms. All of these are pressing concerns indeed, but a deeper issue is the gender-neutral abstraction of their theories which helps to account for the omission of sexuality.

A possible reply at this point might be that sexuality is "omitted" from these theories only in the same sense in which other specific experiences are, such as buying a home, volunteering for political campaigns, racing stock cars, reading novels, or playing musical instruments—for all of these experiences are contained in the pluralistic liberal vision of pursuing the good life as one conceives it. Just as liberalism seeks to maximize for everyone the opportunity to make choices in these various areas, making choices about one's sexuality is also included in the package, even though it is not addressed specifically.

Yet these other desires are different in at least one extremely significant respect. The pursuit of fiction reading, for example, is not connected to an array of social practices that dichotomize novelists and readers as one of the most significant distinctions in our society, in the way that gender is. People do not generally speculate before a child is born whether it will be a reader or a writer. Children are not differentially socialized on the basis of this distinction, nor are readers and writers thought to be biologically destined to relate to one another in specific ways, nor are people judged in virtually every arena of life in terms of whether their behavior and appearance appropriately reflects their status as readers or writers. We do not live in a society in which many authors are coerced by readers to perform acts of fiction against their will. In short, gender is not simply a classificatory concept of biology as well as a social reality; it is a social norm which structures individual subjectivity and social relations to a profound degree, and frequently in inegalitarian ways.

The individual expression of sexual choice as an aspect of the good life is not simply one of many options in specific areas which are open to individuals. Understanding sexuality in this way is so abstract as to be inaccurate, ignoring the influence and impact of ideologies of gender and sexual orientation, as well as race, class, and other social norms of embodiment. My argument is that if justice is one of the goals of theorizing, sexuality must be addressed in terms of oppression and social group differentials. Otherwise women's interests will be neglected, as I have argued is the case in the work of Gauthier and Daniels.

The distributive paradigm does not readily admit issues of sexuality in any clear-cut way. On the descriptive account of health, women are naturally destined to reproduce, but not to be sexually active while avoiding reproduction. How can reproduction be defined as a species-typical function for women, and thus a function worthy of medical support, while women's pursuit of sexual choices apart from reproduction is not defined as a species-typical function? This notion not only categorizes species-typical function arbitrarily, but also reinforces an inegalitarian climate for women by preserving distinct advantages for heterosexual men in their sexual options. In addition, it undermines equality for lesbians, and gay and bisexual men, whose sexuality Boorse treats as dubious at best.

Would it be enough simply to add, for instance, gender and sexual orientation caveats, mandating greater sensitivity to the needs of women and of gay and bisexual men? I think not. These theories direct our attention selectively toward some health-related concerns and away from others, giving no guidance on issues that should be recognized as among the most pressing from the standpoint of justice because of their relation to broader aspects of oppression; and they contribute to the naturalization of socially created health care needs.

In some of the examples cited in this chapter, the concerns of an oppressed group, or the social aspects of an interference with health, are not recognized at all. For example, Gauthier does not discuss personal safety concerns, but most likely would identify them as generally an individual problem, perhaps accidental in some sense, not socially occasioned unless identifiable agencies were directly responsible. Daniels, by contrast, recognizes safe living and working conditions as a health care need, yet he does not address how this issue particularly affects members of oppressed groups, or the social issues involved in rectifying the problem.

Similarly, Daniels's concept of quasi-coerciveness, so usefully applied to the context of the workplace to address the needs and interests of workers, is not extended to the arena of sexuality or reproduction. Ultimately,

Daniels's use of this concept obscures more than it reveals, since this phenomenon is not limited to the context of occupational hazards, but is a pervasive feature of daily life for members of oppressed groups—in fact, is part of the meaning of oppression.[16] Moreover, while Daniels rightly argues that justice in the arena of health requires an equitable distribution of the risk of injury and illness, his work falls far short of conceptualizing what that entails, since he lacks awareness of oppression, social group differentials, and the experiences of specific groups. Indeed, if my discussion of issues in women's health has been successful, it will have shown that his arguments reinscribe certain aspects of a distribution of risk which is inequitable to women.

The descriptive account of health has the admirable aim of avoiding the corruption of medicine with undefended values. Yet it depends on an allegedly pure and untainted medical science which is not critically examined, leaving it vulnerable to the very corruption it seeks to escape. Science is always structured by cultural values, in its historical evolution as well as its current practice. Daniels assigns to medicine the role of safeguarding social justice. This requires integrating egalitarian values such as fostering personal autonomy, which in turn necessitates a thorough critique of the social norms of gender, race, class, and sexuality which are structured into medical theory and practice, along the lines of the work done by the women's health and AIDS movements. The needs, concerns, and demands of oppressed groups ground the recognition that male dominance and institutionalized heterosexism are public health problems, and that preventing these problems requires more than access to health care. It calls for dismantling institutionalized heterosexism and male dominance, a project that requires the participation of every social institution, including medicine.

Epilogue:
Invoke Health and Everyone Jumps

One chilly winter day, Diana, a three-year-old whose grasp of rhetoric exceeds her years, was not in the mood for outdoor play. She drew her preschool teacher aside, asking, "Can we stay inside today? I think my friends will get sick if they go outside now. It's cold!"

In another instance of health rhetoric in daily life, the syndicated columnist Miss Manners addresses the query of a reader baffled by butter knife protocol, wondering whether there are "functional reasons (hygiene, perhaps)" at stake. The columnist responds:

Gentle Reader:

Sometimes Miss Manners thinks she should come up with a list of health considerations to match every single etiquette rule. Nobody seems able to comprehend why decent behavior is needed, but the minute you invoke health, everyone jumps.

She goes on to instruct readers in the proper method for avoiding "a public health threat [posed] by using your own butter knife on the community butter" (Martin 1998, D6).

These moments typify the pervasiveness of health discourse in everyday practical decisions. As Miss Manners suggests, it is a language uniquely capable of moving people to action. In some cases, such as Diana's, the value of health provides an opportune rationale for pursuing one's own self-interested goals. In others, such as the butter knife query, the value of health is pursued for the sake of its apparently inherent and self-justifying correctness (perhaps even when the sought-after outcome is trivial or imperceptible, suggesting the symbolic aspect of health values).

In this book I have been concerned mainly with uses of health discourse which in some way contribute to oppressive beliefs and practices. One may be tempted to oppose the status of health as a central myth in contemporary society, or work to limit its oppressive potential by narrowing its scope. I argue instead that it offers an extremely productive opportunity for pursuing immediate practical goals (such as education for negotiating consent and safer sex, or measures to improve maternal and infant health), as well as egalitarian mythmaking which can ground further action for social change.

To pursue such goals, we must recognize the fundamental connection between "scientific" values as they apply to medicine, and moral-political values and commitments. Epistemic models such as Lisa Heldke and Stephen Kellert's "Objectivity as Responsibility" can assist in this task (1995). Rather than defining objectivity in opposition to subjectivity, they offer an alternative formulation which includes concerns such as the effects of knowledge as it is employed in various contexts. Anyone affected by a diagnosis, an article in bioethics or medicine, a bioethics consultation, or a finding of the Food and Drug Administration must be among those who have a say in evaluating the knowledge produced by these inquiries.

Along these lines, I advocate an anti-oppression model of medical knowledge and care, one that evaluates research, for example, not only on the basis of standard scientific criteria and its usefulness in safe and effective care, but also for its value in eradicating oppressive cultural influences and practices which undermine the health of members of oppressed groups. A material-semiotic understanding of health, illness, and the body itself is needed; we must recognize the inseparability of human biology from human culture and the mutual embeddedness of "scientific" phenomena with the social, the political, and the psychological. Researchers, health care providers, policy makers, and bioethicists must pay greater attention to social group differentials in health, and to issues specific to various groups, as activists have been saying for years.

We should include problems of oppressed groups in research, and include members of those groups as clinicians and researchers. One major avenue toward such inclusiveness is "participatory action research, in which the population of interest is integrally involved in every step of the research process, from problem identification through design conceptualization, implementation, interpretation of findings, and finally outcome evaluation" (Krotoski, Nosek, and Turk 1996, 448). Oppressed groups must be represented in medical fields because of the vital contributions they can make in advancing just science and care. Expertise goes beyond the traditional notion of rigorous professional training and ongoing accomplished practice; experiences related to illness as well as oppression must be a part of the clinical and bioethical knowledge bases. Situated knowledges have much to offer a just medicine.

Information should be transmitted in more accessible ways. Clinicians and researchers must pursue strategies both for sharing their knowledge more fully and effectively with laypersons and for listening to and making use of the information that laypersons can provide, as members of oppressed groups, and as individuals who have a different knowledge of their bodies which should also be heeded in medical contexts. Medical professionals, along with bioethicists, must use their professional status and expertise to oppose oppressive and restrictive policies and to advocate for the interests of oppressed groups.

One strategy for creating the kind of medical climate I have described involves changes in medical education. Practitioners need diversity training that emphasizes respectful treatment for people of diverse cultures, sexual orientations, physical ability levels, and so on. Their training should also include a strong humanities component, providing insights into the political, humanistic, experiential, and ethical aspects of health and medicine (Poirier and Brauner 1988, Segal 1997). The curriculum should provide a thorough study of sexuality from a political and sociocultural perspective, a necessary corrective to the homophobia, erotophobia, and stigmatizing of women's sexualities common in medicine and more broadly.

Another valuable training measure would involve an extensive experiential component in which medical students assume the roles of patients. Although most students will already have experienced patienthood to some degree, incorporating this practice into the curriculum would make a vital statement about the value of that knowledge, and provide opportunities to reflect on its implications for medical practice. Perhaps most important, this training could provide a range of methods for fostering medical self-consciousness in various contexts. This should be coupled with a corresponding respect for the judgments and credibility of laypersons, especially members of oppressed groups who have been denied this respect in many areas of life. Such respect is particularly crucial for survivors of violence.

A related area of transformation is that of agency, the ability of patients to exercise power not only in their own health care and over their own health, but in their lives more generally. The women's health and AIDS movements stress the need for medicine to facilitate rather than undermine the agency of laypersons. Medicine should seek, for example, to foster a sense of control for women. This insight has implications for procedures used in examinations of rape victims as well as in routine gynecological care, the "management" of childbirth, pain relief, and health matters that are related to sexuality in any way. If changes in these areas were to become standard fare in medical training, it is likely that patients would be empowered in other aspects of care as well, which would be an important part of broader social and political empowerment.

Medicine stands as the only remaining shared public discourse that legitimates differential treatment based on one's identity. As the AIDS epidemic has so clearly demonstrated, the power of medical discourse to make people jump can be a dangerous one, particularly for members of oppressed groups. Yet this power cannot be refused or avoided, for just these reasons. It is omnipresent, from playgrounds and breakfast tables to public hospital maternity wards and institutions such as Gay Men's Health Crisis in New York. Medicine must become an arena for social change rather than social control.

Notes

Introduction

1. For discussion, see Marion Banzhaf, Tracy Morgan, and Karen Ramspacher (1990); Shelley Mains and Stephanie Poggi (1990).

2. The book as a whole offers many examples of oppression in the context of health and medicine, and also discusses connections between these examples and other aspects of oppression. Some readers, however, may wish to read a more concentrated argument for this claim. Mab Segrest provides a compelling account of the ways in which racism, classism, sexism, and homophobia are interwoven in U.S. history and contemporary life (1994, 181–246). This work is a valuable starting point for understanding the interaction of these social forces. On the topic of disability, see Susan E. Browne, Debra Connors, and Nanci Stern (1985); Barbara Hillyer (1993); Danuta Krotoski, Margaret Nosek, and Margaret Turk (1996); and Susan Wendell (1996). Gloria Anzaldúa writes of oppression as a lesbian mestiza "border woman" (1987). Angela Davis examines the arenas in which women's oppression has occurred historically, as well as racial and class differences in women's experiences (1981). For Susan Faludi and Susan Sherwin, women's oppression constitutes the backdrop to the themes of an anti-feminist backlash and medical sexism, respectively; both, however, offer concise and persuasive overviews of current manifestations of women's oppression in North America (see Faludi 1991, esp. xiii–xv; Sherwin 1992, esp. 13–26). Linda Tschirhart Sanford and Mary Ellen Donovan address the psychological consequences of patriarchy for women, exploring social institutions such as education, the family, and medicine (1984). In terms of oppression on the basis of sexual orientation, see Warren J. Blumenfeld

(1992), Blumenfeld and Diane Raymond (1988), Loraine Hutchins and Lani Kaahumanu (1991), Craig O'Neill and Kathleen Ritter (1992), James T. Sears (1991), and Elizabeth Reba Weise (1992). These works address many aspects of oppression, as well as the diversity among lesbians, gay men, and bisexuals, and how oppression operates in the context of that diversity.

3. The Combahee River Collective, a group of black feminists, define their political outlook in this way: "We are actively committed to struggling against racial, sexual, heterosexual, and class oppression and see as our particular task the development of integrated analysis and practice based upon the fact that the major systems of oppression are interlocking" (1979, 362). They emphasize that their identity is a central aspect of this political outlook: "We believe that the most profound and potentially the most radical politics come directly out of our own identity, as opposed to working to end somebody else's oppression" (365). See also Shane Phelan (1989).

4. Lisa Heldke and Stephen Kellert persuasively critique the notion of objectivity as detachment, offering an alternative conception of objectivity as responsiveness "to the claims, demands, and criticisms offered by other inquirers" (1995, 363), as well as accountability for the consequences of inquiry. They also provide a useful review of various senses of objectivity.

5. See also Sandra Harding's concept of "traitorous identities" (1991, 288–94).

6. Important examinations of feminist reproductive ethics include Dion Farquhar (1996), Christine Overall (1987), Laura Purdy (1996), and Janice Raymond (1994); also *Hypatia* (1989b). Broader treatments of health care from a feminist perspective include Mary Mahowald (1993), Janice Raymond (1982), and Susan Sherwin's groundbreaking *No Longer Patient* (1992). While Sherwin generally does not invoke the language of justice, her emphasis on the relation between sexist oppression and health care situates her analysis within this framework. Another example is Susan Wolf's *Feminism and Bioethics* (1996), a collection that treats justice as one of many concerns.

7. See Seyla Benhabib (1986), Susan Bordo (1990), Alison Jaggar (1983), Nancy Fraser (1986), and Iris Young (1990).

8. See, for example, Constance Penley (1996).

9. See, for example, Sandra Bartky (1990), Alison M. Jaggar and Susan R. Bordo (1989), and Cindy Patton (1985, 1990).

10. See Gena Corea (1985, 1992), Barbara Duden (1993), Brigitte Jordan (1983), Emily Martin (1987), Ann Oakley (1980), and Barbara Katz Rothman (1982).

11. Useful and provocative examples include Douglas Crimp (1988), Richard Dyer (1991), and Linda Williams (1989).

12. See Nancy Tuana (forthcoming), who argues that "representation does not supersede materiality, nor vice versa."

13. An important body of feminist work questions the value for women of the

framework of justice. A number of useful discussions of, and critical responses to, this work can be found in Claudia Card (1991); see also Joan Tronto (1989). I concur with Susan Moller Okin (1989) and Iris Young (1990) on the potential benefits of the justice framework for women. Young asserts: "The concept of justice is co-extensive with the political" (9). When women's perspectives are integrated into this conceptual framework, I believe it will have great potential to assist in the moral analysis of power relations operating in any area of experience.

14. See John Rawls (1971).

15. See Maria Lugones and Elizabeth Spelman (1983).

16. See Jeffrey Weeks (1977), Morris Kaplan (1997), and Timothy Murphy (1992).

17. Representative examples include Linda Alcoff and Elizabeth Potter (1993), Sandra Harding (1986, 1991), and Alison Jaggar (1983, 1989).

1. Her Body Her Own Worst Enemy

1. A survey of 10,847 women ages fifteen to forty-four was conducted in 1995 by the National Center for Health Statistics (Barbara Vobejda 1997), and 6,748 girls and boys were surveyed by the Commonwealth Fund in 1997 (Judy Mann 1997).

2. See the *Journal of Medicine and Philosophy* special issue, "Women and Medicine" (1982), edited by Caroline Whitbeck. Several authors in this volume, particularly Mary C. Rawlinson, address the pathologization of femaleness. I refer to femaleness as a social construct, not to endorse a notion of "true sex." See Nancy Tuana (forthcoming).

3. Mary Daly's groundbreaking *Gyn/Ecology* (1978) critiques "the Gynecological Culture" and its "imposed totalitarian Heterosexism" (264) and misogyny, identifying medicine as an aspect of patriarchal culture which destroys women's selfhood. Like many feminists, I am deeply indebted to Daly's work. My approach differs from hers, however, in at least two significant ways. First, Daly posits an inherent or essential "Female Self" alienated and undermined by the external forces of patriarchy; while I am also concerned with the erosion of women's selfhood, I do not identify femaleness as the core of women's identity. Second, although Daly critiques medicine as a patriarchal institution, her purpose is to offer a vision of feminism as radical lesbian separatism rather than to work toward the transformation of medicine, as I am attempting to do.

4. I argue that many important concerns related to women's health are obscured by the mainstream medical paradigm. Some readers may wonder whether this position entails claims about intentionality on the part of particular agents. My focus,

however, is on the *effects* of medical epistemology and the disciplinary constraints of mainstream medical discourse; in general, the intentionality of particular agents is not a central concern of this analysis. This approach is in keeping with the view of oppression outlined in my introduction, focusing on the effects of practices, beliefs, and attitudes on a particular social group, rather than on the agency of any deliberate oppressors who may or may not exist.

5. See William Arney (1982), Judith Walzer Leavitt (1986), Barbara Katz Rothman (1982), and Richard Wertz and Dorothy Wertz (1977).

6. Bill Moyers's interviews (1993) with medical researchers and clinicians attest to a growing body of research that demonstrates the importance of these humanistic concerns in diagnosis, treatment, and prognosis. See also Daniel Goleman and Joel Gurin (1993), James Pennebaker (1990), and Christopher Peterson and Lisa Bossio (1991).

7. Carole Warshaw (1994). See also Shelley Bannister (1993) and Lenore Walker (1979) for analyses of the disadvantages battered women face in attempting to voice their concerns within the legal system.

8. The editors of this textbook are to be commended, however, given that others (for example, Danforth and Scott 1986; Rosenwaks, Benjamin, and Stone 1987) fail to include chapters on this important topic.

9. I focus here on the normative aspects of menstrual medicine; however, there are important concerns at an even more basic level. In fact, some feminist critics dispute the very existence of a premenstrual "syndrome," while others advocate a more rigorous conceptualization. Ellen Mitchell and her coauthors find major inconsistencies in definitions of the threshold for severity of PMS symptoms, as well as a lack of uniform symptom typology (1992, 9). Carol Tavris identifies a number of other flaws in standard views of PMS: no evidence of a "biological marker . . . that distinguishes women who have severe premenstrual symptoms from those who do not" (1992, 144); an exaggeration of physiological and psychological differences between women and men, and minimization of the similarities (148–49); an emphasis in the literature on negative aspects of menstruation, while women's reports of positive experiences receive little attention (146); and particularly in the early 1970s no publication of those studies that tended to disconfirm PMS as a widespread phenomenon, a publishing trend that has gradually begun to change (145).

10. See also Sandra Coney (1994) and Michael Martin (1985).

11. See the 1981 World Health Organization Report (Martin 1987, 51), and R. Don Gambrell (1987; cited in Coney 1994, 61).

12. This theme also appears in the literature on hormone replacement therapy in menopause. Sandra Coney includes a sampling of magazine advertisements for hormone supplements and other drugs, one of which displays a smiling couple who appear to be about sixty, with large type proclaiming, "Menrium treats the menopausal symptoms that bother him most" (1994).

13. See Boston Women's Health Book Collective (1992), Wendy Johnson (1996), and Corbett Joan O'Toole (1996).

14. Gloria Steinem cites, for example, "the results of a 150-nation menopause study: negative symptoms *increased* when women went from more to less social mobility and power, but *decreased* when women's power and freedom grew" (1992, 246). See also Ann M. Voda, Myra Dinnerstein, and Sheryl R. O'Donnell (1982).

15. See Dion Farquhar (1996) and Janice Raymond (1994) for contrasting approaches to this topic.

16. See Helen Dewar's report (1996) on related federal legislation in 1996.

17. See, for example, ACT UP/NY Women (1990).

18. Adele Laslie (1982) argues convincingly for this point. More generally, she provides an extremely useful overview of moral issues in childbirth from a feminist perspective.

19. Vrinda Dalmiya and Linda Alcoff argue that the modern epistemological tradition, by defining propositional knowledge as the paradigm of knowledge, excludes women's traditional knowledge. Their chief example is the cultural delegitimation of midwives, whose "practical knowledge" and "experiential knowledge" have been accorded the status of "old wives' tales" (1993, 224).

20. See, for example, Ivan Illich (1977).

2. Physician, Queer Thyself

1. For example, since the early 1980s and continuing through 1996, there has been a steady increase in the number of reported hate crimes against lesbians, gay men, and bisexuals, as well as in the severity of these crimes as measured by the number of offenses committed in a given incident (Fox 1995). The Southern Poverty Law Center reports that reported hate crimes rose from 500 to 2,529, "about 260 percent from 1988 to 1996, according to one count (although these numbers are at least partly accounted for by increased reporting by victims). . . . The figures almost certainly underestimate the number of people attacked," owing to reluctance to report, as well as police failure to classify hate crimes as such (Southern Poverty Law Center 1997, 16).

A 1994 Los Angeles Commission on Human Relations report found that "Gay men topped the list of groups most victimized by hate crimes in Los Angeles County," and "attacks against Gays tended to be more violent than those against other groups" ("Gays Top List" 1994). A study of anti-gay murders in twenty-nine states found them to involve "'extraordinary and horrific violence' of a sort 'fueled by rage and hate,'" and that they are less likely to be solved by police than other homicides ("Group: Gays Killings" 1994). Homophobia on the part of law enforcement as well as defense attorneys, judges, and even prosecutors makes these cases notoriously difficult to prosecute (Minkowitz 1992).

Actual or perceived HIV-positive status is also a risk factor for violence, regardless of sexual orientation. A 1996 National Association of People with AIDS survey of 1,800 people who are HIV positive indicates that "21 percent identified themselves as having experienced violence in their communities because of their HIV status and another 12 percent had been abused in their own homes" (O'Connell 1996, 27).

2. Such commonalities tend to be addressed most often by cultural studies scholars (many of whom I cite in the text), and by activist writers outside the academy, such as ACT UP/NY Women (1990), some of the contributors to Marlene Gerber Fried's *From Abortion to Reproductive Freedom* (1990), and Urvashi Vaid (1995). In the areas of bioethics and social and political theory, Shane Phelan (1989), Susan Sherwin (1992), and Iris Young (1990) are among those who address this connection, though it is not necessarily central to their work, as it is to this analysis.

3. See also Michel Foucault (1980, esp. 42–43) and Shane Phelan (1989, 27–28).

4. At this writing, the Supreme Court has agreed to review a 1990 law imposing "'decency' standards" on the National Endowment for the Arts as a criterion for its grants (Biskupic 1997). Rulings are expected to be issued while this book is in press.

5. In "Policy, Ritual, Purity: Mandatory AIDS Testing," Richard Mohr (1988) argues that mandatory premarital screening for HIV serves a similar symbolic function.

6. See also Gena Corea (1992).

7. Ruth Faden and colleagues provide a strong body of evidence for this claim (1996). They also argue that this treatment of women as "vessels and vectors" occurs in bioethics too, which has focused on the ethical problems of women transmitting the virus to others, rather than on problems related to the research and treatment of women and HIV. See also Cindy Patton (1990).

8. In "Lesbian 'Sex'" (1992), Marilyn Frye provides a critique, both amusing and insightful, of problematic assumptions that structure the individuation and counting of sex acts. She identifies a phallocentric understanding of erotic interactions encoded in the phrase "having sex," resulting in the common perception that lesbians "have sex" less than others. She concludes that this phrase is semantically inappropriate to describe lesbian erotic practice, and advocates the invention of a new vocabulary of lesbian eroticism.

9. See also "Taking Chances with AIDS" (1997).

10. According to the Reverend Lou Sheldon of the Traditional Values Coalition, "They [gays and lesbians] are seeking extra status for a lifestyle which is immoral and a health risk. . . . They should not be working with children, they should not be role models" ("Views on Gay Issues" 1993).

11. See Iris Young's argument that standard usage of the concept of "special interest groups" functions to obscure the appeal to justice in the demands of oppressed groups (1990, 72–74).

12. See Sue Fisher (1986, 7) and Eileen Nechas and Denise Foley (1994, 148–49).

13. See Marilyn Frye's very useful discussion (1983, 1–16).

14. "The sexual unorthodoxy" is Patton's term for the school of theorists also known as the new sex radicals, many of whom are feminist, and most of whom are influenced by poststructuralist or psychoanalytic theorists such as Michel Foucault and Jacques Lacan. Some have identified themselves as "anti–anti-pornography" feminists in response to the 1980s feminist debates on pornography. Two key works in the feminist sexuality debates of this period are Ann Snitow, Christine Stansell, and Sharon Thompson (1983) and Carole S. Vance (1984).

Queer theory includes, for example, the work of many contributors to *The Lesbian and Gay Studies Reader* (Abelove and Halperin, 1993) and to *Inside/Out* (Fuss, 1991). These theorists espouse the designation "queer" for its transgressive value as well as its potential for cutting across standard categorizations of sexuality; they tend to be influenced by European poststructuralist thinking; and many of them work in cultural studies.

Not all of the work being done in queer theory is necessarily compatible with feminism, nor is all feminist sexual theory necessarily gay-affirmative. Furthermore, I must add a cautionary note that the concept of transgression is by no means inherently progressive, insofar as it leaves room for a wide range of nonconsensual, or not fully consensual, sexual practices. My position, however, is that these theoretical stances, used critically, have much to offer a multifactorial analysis of oppression, in medical contexts and elsewhere.

15. Masturbation is "safe" sex not only in the standard sense of avoiding disease, but also in the culturally neglected context of the sexual risks which are particularly imposed on women: sexual violence and unwanted pregnancy. See Linda Singer's critique of "safe sex" rhetoric (1993).

16. This norm helps to explain the otherwise puzzling comment by Cardinal James Hickey of the Washington, D.C., archdiocese, affirming "the fundamental importance of the family for the well-being of society" in response to Elders's masturbation remarks (Marcus 1994).

3. Real Selves

1. See essays by Bridgett Davis, Marian Wright Edelman, and Evelyn White in White's *Black Women's Health Book* (1990); Deborah Bernal (1996); Edward Beards-

ley (1990); Jack Geiger, Harold Luft, and David Mechanic in *The Nation's Health* (Lee, Estes, and Ramsay 1984); and John Lantos, Stephen Thomas, and Sandra Crouse Quinn in *"It Just Ain't Fair": The Ethics of Health Care for African-Americans* (Dula and Goering 1994).

2. See essays by Sheila Battle, Angela Davis, Beverly Smith, Barbara Smith, and Jewelle Gomez in *The Black Women's Health Book* (White 1990); Annette Dula, Leonard Harris, Jean Schensul and Barbara Guest, Evelyn White, and Shafia Monroe in *"It Just Ain't Fair"* (Dula and Goering 1994); Wornie L. Reed, Leonard Syme and Lisa Berkman, and Peter Schnall and Rochelle Kern in *The Sociology of Health and Illness* (Conrad and Kern 1981); and Margaret Nosek (1996b).

3. Troyen Brennan (1991) is an important exception to the norm in bioethics, taking the framework of justice beyond the typical focus on allocation and distribution or the doctor-patient relationship to concerns such as quality of care, various AIDS issues, and doctors' role as policy advocates for patient interests—although he does not address social relations in the broad sense advocated here.

4. This general outlook is shared to varying degrees by much of the recent work in feminist bioethics. See, for example, Susan Sherwin (1992), Susan Wendell (1996), and various contributions to Susan Wolf's *Feminism and Bioethics* (1996). The overall approach of my analysis, however, differs from these works, containing a double emphasis on feminism and sexual inclusiveness rather than focusing primarily on women's perspectives; situating itself within the discourse of justice; and stressing the connectedness of moral, political, and epistemological questions in health and health care.

5. For applications of human connectedness to bioethics, see Hilde Lindemann Nelson and James Lindemann Nelson (1996), Margo Okazawa-Rey (1994), and Mildred Williamson (1994).

6. I am objecting here not to objectivity per se but rather to those constructions of it which regard detachment and neutrality as normative. There are conceptions of objectivity, such as Lisa Heldke and Stephen Kellert's notion of objectivity as responsibility (1995), which are quite compatible with the views defended here.

7. Cf. Lisa Heldke and Stephen Kellert's notion of objectivity as responsibility, which emphasizes relationships among members of the inquiry context (1995).

8. Although I oppose market theories of access, a detailed analysis of Gauthier's conclusion that market access is compatible with justice is outside the scope of this project. I note only that his treatment of this issue is quite cavalier, given the oft-cited statistic of 40 million uninsured Americans (Robert Sherrill 1995, 45). I direct readers interested in this topic to Robert Sherrill's excellent and scathing critique of the role of various market forces (hospitals, the American Medical Association, drug and insurance companies, and health care conglomerates) in the health care system (1995). One point of particular interest is Sherrill's evidence that competing

health maintenance organizations may drive costs up rather than contain them, as Gauthier supposes.

9. I am indebted to Samantha Brennan for her helpful formulation of this point.

10. Cited in Maribeth VanDerWeele (1991).

11. See, for example, Margo Culley and Catherine Portuges (1985), Paulo Freire (1971), John Holt (1982), and A. S. Neill (1964).

12. Sandra Bartky (personal communication).

13. See Mary Field Belenky et al. (1986), Phyllis Chesler (1972), Carol Gilligan (1982), and Gloria Steinem (1992).

14. See discussion in Steinem (1992, 140−45, 212−13).

15. See, for example, essays by Christine Cassel, Annette Dula, John Lantos, Margo Okazawa-Rey, Kristy Woods, and Lauren Jones Young, all in Annette Dula and Sara Goering (1994); also Andrea Lewis and Beverly Smith (1990).

16. A rich body of work has influenced me here. I especially acknowledge Susan Wendell's extremely insightful account of disability, which goes far beyond the usual narrow treatment of the issue in philosophy to address the experience of disability as a moral and epistemic resource for health care reform and broader social change (1996).

17. Daniels believes, however, that his approach is also compatible with other frameworks, such as utilitarianism (1985, 42−48).

18. More recently, in *Seeking Fair Treatment* (1995), Daniels does challenge certain aspects of the system, advocating various reforms in response to broader problems which the AIDS epidemic has dramatized. Although many of these proposed changes would constitute a significant improvement, overall his analysis stays mainly within the limits of the distributive paradigm and of mainstream bioethics, giving little or no attention to matters of social group difference, the moral authority of medicine, or cultural aspects of health and medicine.

19. Daniels (1995) extends the distributive framework to sex education policy for public schools, arguing for the "comprehensive" approach, which includes information on contraception and condom use, rather than an "abstinence-only" framework, which does not. His argument is based on the increasing evidence that comprehensive sex education lowers HIV transmission rates, and thus it is unfair that young people in some communities have access to this safeguard while those in other communities do not. Although this distributive argument is interesting and novel, and again would constitute an improvement if implemented as federal policy, it overlooks those aspects of safer sex practice related to sexual orientation, which I discuss in Chapter 2, and it does not address contraception at all. I take up the latter issue more fully in Chapter 4.

20. An important exception to Daniels's abstract conception of choice is his discussion of "quasi-coerciveness" (a theme I address extensively in Chapter 4) in the context of the occupational choices of individuals. Although "quasi-coerciveness"

is a useful reconceptualization of choice in relation to specific features of the social world, Daniels utilizes this conception only in the context of employment.

21. See Bill Moyers's interview with David Smith, M.D., commissioner of the Texas Department of Health and former chief executive officer and medical director of the innovative Community Oriented Care Program of Parkland Memorial Hospital in Dallas (1993).

22. See Alastair Campbell on giving voice first to those who are worst off (1995), and Mary Mahowald on proportionate representation (1993).

4. Restricted Choices

1. See Steven Schwartzberg's discussion of these themes in the lives of gay men with AIDS (1996).

2. An Environmental Protection Agency task force report indicates a pattern of "environmental racism" in the United States. For example, lead poisoning is higher among African Americans than other groups; areas occupied by blacks and Latinos are more likely than those where whites live to have air pollution levels in excess of federal standards; and American Indians living near waterways may face a higher risk of carcinogens than others (Weisskopf 1992). A 1994 report prepared by the American Wildlife Federation, the African American Environmentalist Association, and the National Association of Neighborhoods finds that in the District of Columbia, "the . . . most heavily African American neighborhoods also are its most polluted, by cars, illegal dumping, leaking oil, sewer overflows and other contamination" (Cohn 1994).

3. Norman Daniels's discussion of cigarette smoking also offers an alternative to this narrow view (1985, 56).

4. See also Peter Breggin (1991), Ivan Illich (1977), and Thomas Szasz (1974).

5. See Tristram Engelhardt's critique of the conflation of species survival with individual health (1976).

6. Boorse argues that reproduction is important in his account of health not so much because of its contribution to the species but because the reproduction of the individual's genes ensures one kind of individual survival (1987, 312). I find this metaphorical argument unpersuasive.

7. See also Carroll Smith-Rosenberg (1985).

8. See Ruth Hubbard (1990), Dierdre Janson-Smith (1980), Brigitte Jordan (1983), and Emily Martin (1987).

9. See also Richard Gelles and Murray Straus (1988, 25–32).

10. See Lenore Walker's discussion of the increasing frequency and severity of violence during a woman's pregnancy and her children's infancy (1979, 105–6).

11. See Gena Corea (1985), Mary Daly (1978), Sheryl Burt Ruzek (1978), and Diana Scully (1980), among many valuable analyses.

12. In *Seeking Fair Treatment,* Daniels (1995) argues for comprehensive sex education as a necessary strategy for reducing HIV transmission. He does not address the importance of contraception for young women, for whom sex has never really been "safe," given a context of sexual violence, patriarchal family control, and interference with reproductive autonomy (see Singer 1993). Nor does he consider gender-related aspects of sex education, such as power imbalances that complicate the ability of young women to negotiate consent and avoid unwanted sex, much less negotiate condom use. To ignore these problems is to leave intact some very problematic aspects of the social context which have a bearing not only on HIV transmission and teen pregnancy but also on gender equality more broadly. Furthermore, while Daniels considers a variety of issues, most of them access-related, he does not address any issues related to abortion.

13. See Warren Blumenfeld (1992), as well as any current issue of the *Lambda Update* newsletter of the Lambda Legal Defense and Education Fund, for useful discussions of these topics.

14. See Craig O'Neill and Kathleen Ritter's discussion of the relationship between sexuality and opportunity or life prospects for lesbians and gay men (1992).

15. In his more recent work, Daniels's call for comprehensive sex education (1995) is an important step for young women, but without careful attention to their distinct interests, it fails to address many of the concerns of this chapter.

16. See Marilyn Frye's essay "Oppression" (1983).

References

Abelove, Michele Aina Barale, and David M. Halperin, eds. 1993. *The Lesbian and Gay Studies Reader*. New York: Routledge.

ACT UP/NY Women & AIDS Book Group, eds. 1990. *Women, AIDS, and Activism*. Boston: South End Press.

Alcoff, Linda, and Elizabeth Potter. 1993. *Feminist Epistemologies*. New York: Routledge.

Alonso, Ana Maria, and Maria Teresa Koreck. 1989. "Silences: 'Hispanics,' AIDS, and Sexual Practices." *Differences* 1(1): 101–24.

Altman, Dennis. 1987. *AIDS in the Mind of America*. Garden City, N.Y.: Anchor Books.

Antonio, Gene. 1988. "Legal Restrictions Are Needed to Control AIDS." In *AIDS: Opposing Viewpoints*, ed. Lynn Hall and Thomas Modl, 128–33. St. Paul, Minn.: Greenhaven Press.

Anzaldúa, Gloria. 1987. *Borderlands/La Frontera: The New Mestiza*. San Francisco: Spinsters/Aunt Lute.

———, ed. 1990. *Making Face, Making Soul*. San Francisco: Spinsters/Aunt Lute.

Apple, Rima D., ed. 1990. *Women, Health, and Medicine in America*. New Brunswick, N.J.: Rutgers University Press.

Arms, Suzanne. 1977. *Immaculate Deception*. New York: Bantam.

Arney, William Ray. 1982. *Power and the Profession of Obstetrics*. Chicago: University of Chicago Press.

Baier, Annette. 1987. "The Need for More than Justice." In *Science, Morality, and Feminist Theory*, ed. Marsha Hanen and Kai Nielsen, 41–56. Calgary: University of Calgary Press.

159

———. 1985. "What Do Women Want in a Moral Theory?" *Nous* 19(1): 53–63.

Bair, Barbara, and Susan E. Cayleff, eds. 1993. *Wings of Gauze: Women of Color and the Experience of Health and Illness.* Detroit: Wayne State University Press.

Baldwin, James. 1978. *Just above My Head.* New York: Dial Press.

Bannister, Shelley A. 1993. "Battered Women Who Kill Their Abusers: Their Courtroom Battles." In *It's a Crime: Women and Justice,* ed. Roslyn Muraskin and Ted Alleman, 316–33. Englewood Cliffs, N.J.: Regents/Prentice Hall.

Banzhaf, Marion, Tracy Morgan, and Karen Ramspacher. 1990. "Reproductive Rights and AIDS: The Connections." In *Women, AIDS, and Activism,* ed. ACT UP/NY Women's Book Group, 199–209. Boston: South End Press.

Baron-Faust, Rita. 1989. "Why Doctors Mistreat Women." *Redbook* May: 114–15, 191–95.

Bart, Pauline, and Patricia H. O'Brien. 1985. *Stopping Rape: Successful Survival Strategies.* New York: Pergamon Press.

Bart, Pauline, and Diana Scully. 1973. "A Funny Thing Happened on the Way to the Orifice: Women in Gynecology Textbooks." *American Journal of Sociology* 78: 1045.

Bartky, Sandra Lee. 1990. *Femininity and Domination: Studies in the Phenomenology of Oppression.* New York: Routledge.

Battle, Sheila. 1990. "Moving Targets: Alcohol, Crack, and Black Women." In White, 251–56.

Beardsley, Edward H. 1990. "Race as a Factor in Health." In Apple, 121–39.

Beauchamp, Tom L., and James F. Childress. 1979. *Principles of Biomedical Ethics.* New York: Oxford University Press.

Belenky, Mary Field, Blythe McVicker Clinchy, Nancy Rule Goldberger, and Jill Mattuck Tarule. 1986. *Women's Ways of Knowing.* New York: Basic Books.

Bell, Nora K. 1989. "What Setting Limits May Mean." *Hypatia* 4(2): 169–78.

Benhabib, Seyla. 1986. "The Generalized and the Concrete Other: The Kohlberg-Gilligan Controversy and Feminist Theory." *Praxis International* 5(4): 402–24.

Bennett-Haigney, Lisa. 1997. "Welfare Bill Further Endangers Domestic Violence Survivors." *National Organization for Women Times* 29(1): 5.

Bernal, Deborah L. 1996. "The Perspective of Ethnicity on Women's Health and Disability." In Krotoski, Nosek, and Turk, 57–61.

Biskupic, Joan. 1997. "Judges to Rule on 'Decency' Standards for Arts Funding." *Washington Post* November 27: A4.

Blumenfeld, Warren J., ed. 1992. *Homophobia.* Boston: Beacon Press.

Blumenfeld, Warren J., and Diane Raymond. 1988. *Looking at Gay and Lesbian Life.* New York: Philosophical Library.

Boodman, Sandra G. 1997. "Poor Women Report High Level of Abuse." *Washington Post, "Health"* May 20: 5.

———. 1993. "The Dearth of Abortion Doctors." *Washington Post, "Health"* April 20: 5.

Boorse, Christopher. 1987. "Concepts of Health." In *Health Care Ethics: An Intro-*

duction, ed. Donald VanDeVeer and Tom Regan, 359–93. Philadelphia: Temple University Press.

———. 1981. "On the Distinction between Disease and Illness." In *Medicine and Moral Philosophy,* ed. Marshall Cohen, Thomas Nagel, and Thomas Scanlon, 3–22. Princeton: Princeton University Press.

———. 1976. "What a Theory of Mental Health Should Be." *Journal for the Theory of Social Behavior* 6(1):61–84.

Booth, William. 1993. "In Rural Areas, AIDS Patients Find Little Compassion or Health Care." *Washington Post* June 13:A21.

Bordo, Susan R. 1990. "Feminism, Postmodernism, and Gender-Scepticism." In *Feminism/Postmodernism,* ed. Linda Nicholson, 133–56. New York: Routledge.

Bosk, Charles L., and Joel E. Frader. 1991. "AIDS and Its Impact on Medical Work: The Culture and Politics of the Shop Floor." In *A Disease of Society: Cultural and Institutional Responses to AIDS,* ed. Dorothy Nelkin, David P. Willis, and Scott V. Parris, 150–71. Cambridge: Cambridge University Press.

Boston Women's Health Book Collective. 1992. *The New Our Bodies, Ourselves: A Book by and for Women.* New York: Simon & Schuster/Touchstone.

Bowker, Lee H. 1986. *Ending the Violence.* Holmes Beach, Fla.: Learning Publications.

Breggin, Peter R. 1991. *Toxic Psychiatry.* New York: St. Martin's Press.

Brennan, Troyen. 1991. *Just Doctoring: Medical Ethics in the Liberal State.* Berkeley: University of California Press.

Brighton Women and Science Group, ed. 1980. *Alice Through the Microscope: The Power of Science over Women's Lives.* London: Virago.

Brown, David. 1997. "Evidence Mounts in Favor of 'Triple Therapy' against AIDS Virus." *Washington Post, "Health"* February 4:13.

———. 1994. "20-Year Rise in Caesarean Deliveries Appears to Have Stopped." *Washington Post* May 19:A26.

Browne, Susan E., Debra Connors, and Nanci Stern. 1985. *With the Power of Each Breath: A Disabled Women's Anthology.* Pittsburgh: Cleis Press.

Buchanan, Allen. 1981. "Justice: A Philosophical Review." In *Justice and Health Care,* ed. Earl E. Shelp, 3–21. Boston: D. Reidel.

Bulkin, Elly, Minnie Bruce Pratt, and Barbara Smith. 1984. *Yours in Struggle: Three Feminist Perspectives on Anti-Semitism and Racism.* Brooklyn: Long Haul Press.

Byron, Peg. 1991. "HIV: The National Scandal." *Ms.* 1(4):24–29.

Campbell, Alastair V. 1995. *Health as Liberation: Medicine, Theology, and the Quest for Justice.* Cleveland: Pilgrim Press.

Card, Claudia, ed. 1991. *Feminist Ethics.* Lawrence: University Press of Kansas.

Carter, Erica, and Simon Watney, eds. 1989. *Taking Liberties: AIDS and Cultural Politics.* London: Serpents Tail, in association with the Institute of Contemporary Arts.

Carter, George M. 1992. *ACT UP, the AIDS War, and Activism. Open Magazine Pamphlet Series* 15. Westfield, N.J.: Open Media.

Cartwright, Peter S. 1988. "Sexual Violence." In *Novak's Textbook of Gynecology,* 11th ed., Howard W. Jones III, Anne Colston Wentz, and Lonnie S. Burnett, 525–33. Baltimore: Williams & Wilkins.

Cassel, Christine. 1994. "Commentary." In Dula and Goering, 120–22.

"CDC Wrestles with 'Post Exposure' HIV Therapy." 1997. *Washington Blade* August 1:27.

Chesler, Phyllis. 1972. *Women and Madness.* New York: Avon Books.

Chibbaro, Lou, Jr. 1994. "Out-of-Court Settlement in Philadelphia Case." *Washington Blade* March 25:29.

Chrisler, Joan C. 1993. "Whose Body Is It Anyway? Psychological Effects of Fetal-Protection Policies." In *It's a Crime: Women and Justice,* ed. Roslyn Muraskin and Ted Alleman, 285–90. Englewood Cliffs, N.J.: Regents/Prentice Hall.

Christensen, C., A. King-Meltzer, and B. Feltzer. 1991. "Medical Students' Reactions to AIDS: The Influence of Patient Characteristics on Hypothetical Treatment Decisions." *Teaching and Learning in Medicine* 3:138–42.

Churchill, Larry R. 1987. *Rationing Health Care in America: Perceptions and Principles of Justice.* Notre Dame: University of Notre Dame Press.

Cohen, Sharon. 1990. "Ban on Fertile Women Stirs Job Bias Battle." *Chicago Sun-Times* October 7.

Cohn, D'Vera. 1994. "Blacks Bear Brunt of D.C.'s Pollution." *Washington Post* June 19:B1, 3.

Colburn, Don. 1996. "Question Helps Identify Domestic Violence Cases." *Washington Post, "Health"* July 9:5.

———. 1994. "Domestic Violence: AMA President Decries 'A Major Public Health Problem.'" *Washington Post, "Health"* June 28:10–12.

Combahee River Collective. 1979. "A Black Feminist Statement." In *Capitalist Patriarchy and the Case for Socialist Feminism,* ed. Zillah R. Eisenstein, 362–72. New York: Monthly Review Press.

"Comments after Speech at the U.N." 1994. *Washington Post* March 10:A12.

Coney, Sandra. 1994. *The Menopause Industry: How the Medical Establishment Exploits Women.* Alameda, Calif.: Hunter House.

Conrad, Peter, and Rochelle Kern, eds. 1981. *The Sociology of Health and Illness: Critical Perspectives.* New York: St. Martin's Press.

Corea, Gena. 1992. *The Invisible Epidemic: The Story of Women and AIDS.* New York: HarperCollins.

———. 1985. *Hidden Malpractice: How American Medicine Mistreats Women.* New York: Harper & Row.

"Corrections Concerning Post-exposure Therapy." 1997. *Washington Blade* August 15:26.

Crawford, Robert. 1984. "A Cultural Account of 'Health': Control, Release, and the Social Body." In *Issues of the Political Economy of Health Care,* ed. John McKinlay, 60–103. New York: Tavistock Publications, in association with Methuen.

Crimp, Douglas, ed. 1988. *AIDS: Cultural Analysis, Cultural Activism.* Cambridge: MIT Press.

Culley, Margo, and Catherine Portuges, eds. 1985. *Gendered Subjects.* Boston: Routledge.

Dalmiya, Vrinda, and Linda Alcoff. 1993. "Are 'Old Wives' Tales' Justified?" In *Feminist Epistemologies,* ed. Linda Alcoff and Elizabeth Potter, 217–44. New York: Routledge.

Daly, Mary. 1978. *Gyn/Ecology: The Metaethics of Radical Feminism.* Boston: Beacon Press.

Dan, Alice J., ed. 1994. *Reframing Women's Health: Multidisciplinary Research and Practice.* Thousand Oaks, Calif.: Sage Publications.

Dan, Alice J., and Linda L. Lewis, eds. 1992. *Menstrual Health in Women's Lives.* Urbana: University of Illinois Press.

Danforth, David N., and James R. Scott, eds. 1986. *Obstetrics and Gynecology,* 5th ed. Philadelphia: Lippincott.

Daniels, Norman. 1995. *Seeking Fair Treatment: From the AIDS Epidemic to National Health Care Reform.* New York: Oxford University Press.

———. 1985. *Just Health Care.* Cambridge: Cambridge University Press.

Davis, Angela Y. 1994. "Surrogates and Outcast Mothers: Racism and Reproductive Politics." In Dula and Goering, 40–55.

———. 1990. "Sick and Tired of Being Sick and Tired: The Politics of Black Women's Health." In White, 18–26.

———. 1981. *Women, Race, and Class.* New York: Vintage Books.

Davis, Bridgett M. 1990. "Speaking of Grief: Today I Feel Real Low, I Hope You Understand." In White, 219–25.

Davis, Karen. 1984. "Health Care of Low Income Families." In Lee, Estes, and Ramsay, 55–62.

Davis, Kathy. 1988. "Paternalism under the Microscope." In *Gender and Discourse: The Power of Talk,* ed. Alexandra Todd and Sue Fisher, 19–54. Norwood, N.J.: Ablex.

Deming, Barbara. 1985. *A Humming under My Feet: A Book of Travail.* London: Women's Press.

Denenberg, Risa. 1993. "Gynecological Considerations in the Primary-Care Setting." In *Until the Cure: Caring for Women with HIV,* ed. Ann Kurth, 35–46. New Haven: Yale University Press.

Dewar, Helen. 1996. "AIDS Testing Compromise Is Reached." *Washington Post* May 5:A9.

Dickman, Robert L. 1983. "Operationalizing Respect for Persons: A Qualitative Aspect of the Right to Health Care". In *In Search of Equity: Health Needs and the Health Care System,* ed. Ronald Bayer, Arthur Caplan, and Norman Daniels, 161–82. New York: Plenum Press.

Dobash, R. Emerson, and Russell Dobash. 1979. *Violence against Wives: A Case against the Patriarchy.* New York: Free Press.

"Doctors Balk at Treating AIDS Patients." 1992. *Chicago Tribune* March 22.

Dreifus, Claudia. 1977. *Seizing Our Bodies: The Politics of Women's Health.* New York: Vintage Books.

Duberman, Martin. 1991. *Cures: A Gay Man's Odyssey.* New York: Dutton.

Duden, Barbara. 1993. *Disembodying Women: Perspectives on Pregnancy and the Unborn.* Cambridge: Harvard University Press.

Dula, Annette, and Sara Goering, eds. 1994. *"It Just Ain't Fair: The Ethics of Health Care for African-Americans.* Westport, Conn.: Praeger.

Dyer, Richard. 1991. "Believing in Fairies: The Author and The Homosexual." In Fuss, 185–201.

Eberly, David. 1992. "Homophobia, Censorship, and the Arts." In Blumenfeld, 205–16.

Eckholm, Erik. 1991. "Health Benefits Found to Deter Job Switching." *New York Times* September 26: A1, 13.

Edelman, Marian Wright. 1990. "The Black Family in America." In White, 128–48.

Ehrenreich, Barbara, and John Ehrenreich. 1970. *The American Health Empire: Power, Profits, and Politics.* New York: Random House.

Eisenstein, Zillah R., ed. 1979. *Capitalist Patriarchy and the Case for Socialist Feminism.* New York: Monthly Review Press.

Engelhardt, Tristram. 1976. "Ideology and Etiology." *Journal of the Philosophy of Medicine* 1:264.

Erlanger, Stephen. 1989. "Horror at Home: The Tragedy of Family Violence." *Family Circle* April 4:78–83.

"Estimated Number of Children Born with AIDS Transmitted by Mothers." 1997. *Washington Post, "Health"* January 7:5.

"Facts about Limitations on Abortion Funding." 1990. *NewsNOW* (West Suburban Chapter, National Organization for Women, Illinois) January.

Faden, Ruth, Nancy Kass, and Deven McGraw. 1996. "Women as Vessels and Vectors: Lessons from the HIV Epidemic." In Wolf, 252–81.

Faludi, Susan. 1991. *Backlash: The Undeclared War against American Women.* New York: Crown.

Farquhar, Dion. 1996. *The Other Machine: Discourse and Reproductive Technologies.* New York: Routledge.

Fee, Elizabeth, ed. 1983. *Women and Health: The Politics of Sex in Medicine.* Farmingdale, N.Y.: Baywood Publishing Company.

Fee, Elizabeth, and Daniel M. Fox, eds. 1988. *AIDS: The Burdens of History.* Berkeley: University of California Press.

Ferguson, Warren J. 1994. "The Physician's Responsibility to Medically Underserved Poor People." In Dula and Goering, 123–33.

Figlio, Karl. 1983. "Chlorosis and Chronic Disease in Nineteenth-Century Britain: The Social Constitution of Somatic Illness in a Capitalist Society." In Fee, 213–41.

Fisher, Sue. 1986. *In the Patient's Best Interest: Women and the Politics of Medical Decisions*. New Brunswick, N.J.: Rutgers University Press.

Foucault, Michel. 1980. *The History of Sexuality*, vol. 1, *An Introduction*. New York: Vintage Books. (Trans. *Histoire de la sexualité*, 1, *La volonté de savoir*. Paris: Gallimard, 1976.)

———. 1979. *Discipline and Punish: The Birth of the Prison*. New York: Vintage Books. (Trans. *Surveiller et punir: naissance de la prison*. [Paris]: Gallimard, 1975.)

———. 1975. *The Birth of the Clinic: An Archaeology of Medical Perception*. New York: Vintage Books. (Trans. *Naissance de la Clinique: une archéologie du regard medical*. Paris: Presses Universitaires de France, 1963.)

Fox, Sue. 1995. "In 1994, Anti-Gay Violence Increased Slightly." *Washington Blade* March 10:35.

Fraser, Nancy. 1986. "Toward a Discourse Ethic of Solidarity." *Praxis International* 5.4 (January):425–29.

Freire, Paulo. 1971. *Pedagogy of the Oppressed*. New York: Herder and Herder. (Trans. *Pedagogio del oprimido*. Montivideo: Tierra Nueva, 1970.)

Fried, Marlene Gerber, ed. 1990. *From Abortion to Reproductive Freedom: Transforming a Movement*. Boston: South End Press.

Frye, Marilyn. 1992. *Willful Virgin: Essays in Feminism, 1976–1992*. Freedom, Calif.: Crossing Press.

———. 1983. *The Politics of Reality: Essays in Feminist Theory*. Trumansburg, N.Y.: Crossing Press.

Fuss, Diana, ed. 1991. *Inside Out*. New York: Routledge.

Gauthier, David P. 1986. *Morals by Agreement*. Oxford: Clarendon Press.

———. 1983. "Unequal Need: A Problem of Equity in Access to Health Care." In *Securing Access to Health Care: The Ethical Implications of Differences in the Availability of Health Services*, vol. 2, *Appendices: Sociocultural and Philosophical Studies*. Washington, D.C.: President's Commission for the Study of Ethical Problems in Medicine and Biomedical and Behavioral Research, Government Printing Office, 179–205.

"Gays Top List of Hate Crime Victims in L.A." 1994. *Washington Blade* June 17:10.

Geiger, H. Jack. 1984. "Inequities in Health and Health Care." In Lee, Estes, and Ramsay, 469–72.

Gelles, Richard J., and Murray A. Straus. 1988. *Intimate Violence: The Causes and Consequences of Abuse in the American Family*. New York: Simon & Schuster/ Touchstone.

Gill, Carol J. 1996. "Becoming Visible: Personal Health Experiences of Women with Disabilities." In Krotoski, Nosek, and Turk, 5–15.

Gilligan, Carol. 1982. *In a Different Voice*. Cambridge: Harvard University Press.

Glazer, Sarah. 1994. "IQ at a Glance." *Washington Post, "Health"* June 7:13–15.

Godec, Mark S. 1993. "Your Final 30 Days Free." *Washington Post* May 2:C3.

Goleman, Daniel, and Joel Gurin, eds. 1993. *Mind, Body Medicine: How to Use Your Mind for Better Health*. Yonkers, N.Y.: Consumer Reports Books.

Gomez, Jewelle, and Barbara Smith. 1990. "Taking the Home Out of Homo-
phobia: Black Lesbian Health." In White, 198–213.
Goodman, Gerre, George Lakey, Judy Lashof, and Erica Thorne. 1983. *No Turning
Back: Lesbian and Gay Liberation of the '80s.* Philadelphia: New Society Publishers.
"Group: Gays Killings More Brutal." 1994. *Washington Post* December 21:A2.
Grover, Jan Zita. 1988. "AIDS: Keywords." In Crimp, 17–30.
Haire, Doris. 1972. *The Cultural Warping of Childbirth: A Special Report.* Minne-
apolis: International Childbirth Education Association.
Haraway, Donna J. 1997. *Modest Witness@Second Millennium.FemaleMan Meets
OncoMouse(tm) Feminism and Technoscience.* New York: Routledge.
Harding, Sandra G. 1991. *Whose Science? Whose Knowledge? Thinking from Women's
Lives.* Ithaca: Cornell University Press.
———. 1986. *The Science Question in Feminism.* Ithaca: Cornell University Press.
Harris, Leonard. 1994. "Epilogue." In Dula and Goering, 264–67.
Heise, Lori L. 1994. "Gender-Based Abuse: The Global Epidemic." In Dan,
233–50.
Heldke, Lisa M., and Stephen H. Kellert. 1995. "Objectivity as Responsibility."
Metaphilosophy 26(4):360–78.
Hendrickson, Paul. 1993. "Dr. Elders's Prescription for Battle." *Washington Post*
February 16:D1.
Hillyer, Barbara. 1993. *Feminism and Disability.* Norman: University of Oklahoma
Press.
"HMO Study Questions Operations." 1993. *Washington Post* May 12.
Holt, John Caldwell. 1982. *How Children Fail.* New York: Delta/Seymour Law-
rence.
hooks, bell. 1992. *Black Looks: Race and Representation.* Boston: South End
Press.
———. 1984. *Feminist Theory: From Margin to Center.* Boston: South End Press.
Hubbard, Ruth. 1990. *The Politics of Women's Biology.* New Brunswick, N.J.:
Rutgers University Press.
Hutchins, Loraine, and Lani Kaahumanu, eds. 1991. *Bi Any Other Name: Bisexual
People Speak Out.* Boston: Alyson Publications.
Hypatia. 1989a. Special Issue: Feminist Ethics and Medicine. 4(2).
———. 1989b. Special Issue: Ethics and Reproduction. 4(3).
Illich, Ivan. 1977. *Medical Nemesis: The Expropriation of Health.* New York: Bantam
Books.
Jaggar, Alison M. 1989. "Love and Knowledge: Emotion in Feminist Episte-
mology." In *Women, Knowledge, and Reality: Explorations in Feminist Philosophy,*
ed. Ann Garry and Marilyn Pearsall, 129–55. Boston: Unwin Hyman.
———. 1983. *Feminist Politics and Human Nature.* Totowa, N.J.: Rowman & Al-
lanheld.
Jaggar, Alison M., and Susan R. Bordo, eds. 1989. *Gender/Body/Knowledge: Feminist*

Reconstructions of Being and Knowing. New Brunswick, N.J.: Rutgers University Press.

Janson-Smith, Deirdre. 1980. "Sociobiology: So What?" In Brighton Women, 62–86.

Johnson, Wendy. 1997. "Health Data: Its Depth, Dearth." *Washington Blade* August 1:1, 27.

———. 1996. "Doctors Need Dose of Education, Group Asserts." *Washington Blade* September 27:33.

Jones, Howard W., III, Anne Colston Wentz, and Lonnie S. Burnett. 1988. *Novak's Textbook of Gynecology,* 11th ed. Baltimore: Williams & Wilkins.

Jordan, Brigitte. 1983. *Birth in Four Cultures: A Cross-Cultural Investigation of Childbirth in Yucatan, Holland, Sweden, and the United States.* Montreal: Eden Press.

Journal of Medicine and Philosophy. 1982. Special Issue: Women and Medicine 7(2).

Kaplan, Morris B. 1997. *Sexual Justice: Democratic Citizenship and the Politics of Desire.* New York: Routledge.

Katz, Jonathan. 1976. *Gay American History: Lesbians and Gay Men in the USA.* New York: Avon Books.

Kayal, Philip M. 1993. *Bearing Witness: Gay Men's Health Crisis and the Politics of AIDS.* Boulder: Westview.

Keen, Lisa. 1997. "Slip in Concern?" *Washington Blade* September 11:27.

———. 1996. "AMA Urges Doctors to 'Recognize' Gay Patients." *Washington Blade* May 3:19.

Kestenbaum, Victor, ed. 1982. *The Humanity of the Ill: Phenomenological Perspectives.* Knoxville: University of Tennessee Press.

Killion, Cheryl M. 1990. "Service without Subservience: Reflections of a Registered Nurse." In White, 240–50.

Kinch, Robert A. 1974. "Response to Kaiser and Kaiser." *American Journal of Obstetrics and Gynecology* 120:664.

Knight, Jerry. 1994. "Adding Fuel to the Smoking Fight." *Washington Post* April 19:C1, 2.

Krotoski, Danuta M., Margaret A. Nosek, and Margaret A. Turk, eds. 1996. *Women with Physical Disabilities: Achieving and Maintaining Health and Well-Being.* Baltimore: Paul H. Brookes.

The Lambda Update (Newsletter of Lambda Legal Defense and Education Fund). New York.

Langone, John. 1985. "AIDS." *Discover* 6.12 (December):27–52.

Lantos, John D. 1994. "Disparities in Access and Health Status: An Ethical Issue: Race, Prenatal Care, and Infant Mortality." In Dula and Goering, 67–74.

Laslie, Adele. 1982. "Ethical Issues in Childbirth. *Journal of Medicine and Philosophy* 7(2):179–95.

Leavitt, Judith Walzer. 1986. *Brought to Bed: Childbearing in America, 1750 to 1950.* New York: Oxford University Press.

Lee, Philip R., Carroll L. Estes, and Nancy B. Ramsay, eds. 1984. *The Nation's Health*, 2d ed. San Francisco: Boyd & Fraser.

Leonard, Zoe. 1990. "Lesbians in the AIDS Crisis." In ACT UP, 113–18.

Levi, Jeffrey. 1986. "Public Health and the Gay Perspective: Creating a Basis for Trust." In *AIDS: Facts and Issues,* ed. Victor Gong and Norman Rudnick, 179–88. New Brunswick, N.J.: Rutgers University Press.

Lewis, Andrea, and Beverly Smith. 1990. "Looking at the Total Picture: A Conversation with Health Activist Beverly Smith." In White, 172–81.

Lewis, Linda L. 1992. "PMS and Progesterone: The Ongoing Controversy." In Dan and Lewis, 61–72.

Lifton, Betty Jean. 1979. *Lost and Found: The Adoption Experience.* New York: Dial Press.

Lorde, Audre. 1984. "An Open Letter to Mary Daly." In *Sister Outsider: Essays and Speeches.* Trumansburg, N.Y.: Crossing Press, 66–71.

Luft, Harold S. 1984. "Poverty and Health." In Lee, Estes, and Ramsay, 473–79.

Lugones, Maria C. 1991. "On the Logic of Pluralist Feminism." In Card, 35–44.

———. 1990. "Hablando Cara a Cara/Speaking Face to Face: An Exploration of Ethnocentric Racism." In *Making Face, Making Soul: Haciendo Caras, Creative and Critical Perspectives by Women of Color,* ed. Gloria Anzaldua, 46–54. San Francisco: Aunt Lute Foundation Books.

Lugones, Maria C., and Elizabeth V. Spelman. 1983. "Have We Got a Theory for You! Feminist Theory, Cultural Imperialism, and the Demand for 'The Woman's Voice.'" *Women's Studies International Forum* 6(6): 573–81.

MacIntyre, Alasdair. 1981. *After Virtue.* Notre Dame: University of Notre Dame Press.

Macklin, Ruth. 1994. *Surrogates and Other Mothers: The Debates over Assisted Reproduction.* Philadelphia: Temple University Press.

Mahowald, Mary Briody. 1993. *Women and Children in Health Care: An Unequal Majority.* New York: Oxford University Press.

Mains, Shelley, and Stephanie Poggi. 1990. "'Together We Will Get Somewhere': Working Together for Lesbian/Gay Liberation and Reproductive Freedom." In Fried, 281–90.

Mann, Judy. 1997. "A Perilous Age for Girls." *Washington Post* October 10: E3.

———. 1994. "Elections Do Make a Difference." *Washington Post* May 20: E3.

Marcus, Ruth. 1994. "President Clinton Fires Elders." *Washington Post* December 10: A1, 12.

Martin, Emily. 1987. *The Woman in the Body.* Boston: Beacon Press.

Martin, Judith. 1998. "Butter Safe . . . " *Washington Post* February 4: D6.

Martin, Michael. 1985. "Malady and Menopause." *Journal of Medicine and Philosophy* 10(4): 329–37.

McClory, Robert. 1991. "HIV's Neglected Victims: Women and Children Last." *Chicago Reader* February 1.

McCullough, Laurence V. 1981. "Justice and Health Care: Historical Perspectives and Precedents." In Shelp, 51–71.

Mechanic, David. 1984. "Inequality, Health Status, and the Delivery of Health Services in the United States." In Lee, Estes, and Ramsay, 488–97.

Merton, Vanessa. 1996. "Ethical Obstacles to the Participation of Women in Biomedical Research." In Wolf, 216–51.

Minkowitz, Donna. 1992. "It's Still Open Season on Gays." *The Nation* March 23: 368–70.

"Minnesota Dentist Fined for Denying Treatment to AIDS Patient." 1992. *Chicago Tribune* March 22.

Mitchell, Ellen S., Martha J. Lentz, Nancy F. Woods, Kathryn Lee, and Diana Taylor. 1992. "Methodological Issues in the Definition of Premenstrual Syndrome." In Dan and Lewis, 7–14.

Mohr, Richard. 1998. "Anti-Gay Stereotypes." In *Race, Class, and Gender in the United States: An Integrated Study,* 4th ed., ed. Paula S. Rothenberg, 458–65. New York: St. Martin's Press.

———. 1988. *Gays/Justice.* New York: Columbia University Press.

Morgan, Kathryn. 1997. "Permissibility of Physical Contact between Physicians and Patients." American Philosophical Association Conferences, Pacific Division, Berkeley, March.

Moyers, Bill. 1993. *Healing and the Mind.* New York: Doubleday.

Murphy, Timothy F. 1994. *Ethics in an Epidemic: AIDS, Morality, and Culture.* Berkeley : University of California Press.

———. 1993. "Testimony." In *Writing AIDS,* ed. Timothy F. Murphy and Suzanne Poirier, 306–20. New York: Columbia University Press.

———. 1992. "Redirecting Sexual Orientation: Techniques and Justifications." *Journal of Sex Research* 29:503–23.

———. 1991. "No Time for an AIDS Backlash." *Hastings Center Report* March/April.

———. 1988. "Is AIDS a Just Punishment?" *Journal of Medical Ethics* 14:154–60.

Murphy-Lawless, Jo. 1988. "The Obstetric View of Feminine Identity: A Nineteenth-Century Case History of the Use of Forceps on Unmarried Women in Ireland." In Todd and Fisher, 177–98.

Nagel, Thomas. 1986. *The View from Nowhere.* Oxford: Oxford University Press.

Native American Women's Health Education Resource Center. 1993. "Native American Women Uncover Norplant Abuses." *Ms.* September/October:69.

Nechas, Eileen, and Denise Foley. 1994. *Unequal Treatment: What You Don't Know about How Women Are Mistreated by the Medical Community.* New York: Simon and Schuster.

Neill, A. S. 1964. *Summerhill.* New York: Hart.

Nelkin, Dorothy, David P. Willis, and Scott V. Parris, eds. 1991. *A Disease of Society: Cultural and Institutional Responses to AIDS.* Cambridge: Cambridge University Press.

Nelson, Hilde Lindemann, and James Lindemann Nelson. 1996. "Justice in the Allocation of Health Care Resources: A Feminist Account." In Wolf, 351–70.

"New Study Finds High Rate of Birth Control Failures." 1989. *Chicago Sun-Times* July 13:A1, 18.

Nicholson, Heather J. 1991. "Girls into Science." *Chicago Tribune* October 6:6.

Nicholson, Linda. 1990. *Feminism/Postmodernism*. New York: Routledge.

Norwood, Christopher. 1985. "Terata." *Mother Jones* January:15–21.

Nosek, Margaret. 1996a. "Sexual Abuse of Women with Physical Disabilities." In Krotoski, Nosek, and Turk, 153–73.

———. 1996b. "Wellness among Women with Physical Disabilities." In Krotoski, Nosek, and Turk, 17–33.

Nozick, Robert. 1974. *Anarchy, State, and Utopia*. New York: Basic Books.

Oakley, Ann. 1980. *Women Confined: Towards a Sociology of Childbirth*. New York: Schocken Books.

O'Connell, Brian. 1996. "Report Addresses Violence against PWAs." *Washington Blade* April 12:27.

Okazawa-Rey, Margo. 1994. "Grandparents Who Care: An Empowerment Model of Health Care." In Dula and Goering, 221–33.

Okie, Susan. 1997. "Panel Asserts Politics Hurts AIDS Fight." *Washington Post* February 14:A1, 8.

Okin, Susan Moller. 1989. *Justice, Gender, and the Family*. New York: Basic Books.

O'Neill, Craig, and Kathleen Ritter. 1992. *Coming Out Within*. San Francisco: Harper.

O'Toole, Corbett Joan. 1996. "Disabled Lesbians: Challenging Monocultural Constructs." In Krotoski, Nosek, and Turk, 135–51.

Overall, Christine. 1989. "The Politics of Communities: A Review of H. Tristram Engelhardt Jr.'s *The Foundations of Bioethics*." *Hypatia* 4(2):179–85.

———. 1987. *Ethics and Human Reproduction*. Boston: Allen & Unwin.

Parsons, Christi. 1990. "Abuse of Women More Than Meets Eye, Doctors Learn." *Chicago Tribune* August 26:2C.

Patton, Cindy. 1990. "Why We Can't Get Women and AIDS on the Agenda." *Z* 3(12):99–103.

———. 1985. *Sex and Germs*. Boston: South End Press.

Pellegrino, Edmund D. 1982. "Being Ill and Being Healed: Some Reflections on the Grounding of Medical Morality." In Kestenbaum, 157–66.

Penley, Constance. 1996. "From NASA to the 700 Club (with a Detour through Hollywood): Cultural Studies and the Public Sphere." In *Disciplinarity and Dissent in Cultural Studies,* ed. Cary Nelson and Dilip Parameshwar Gaonkar, 235–50. New York: Routledge.

Pennebaker, James. 1990. *Opening Up*. New York: William Morrow.

Perrow, Charles, and Mauro F. Guillen. 1990. *The AIDS Disaster*. New Haven: Yale University Press.

Peterson, Christopher, and Lisa M. Bossio. 1991. *Health and Optimism*. New York: Free Press.

Phelan, Shane. 1989. *Identity Politics: Lesbian Feminism and the Limits of Community.* Philadelphia: Temple University Press.

Plumb, Marj. 1996. "Close Call Is Hard Reminder of Medical Reality." *Washington Blade* June 7:55.

Poirier, Suzanne. 1990. "Women's Reproductive Health." In Apple, 217–45.

Poirier, Suzanne, and Daniel J. Brauner. 1988. "Ethics and the Daily Language of Medical Discourse." *Hastings Center Report* 18.4 (August/September):5–9.

Poore, Grace, director. 1996. *Voices Heard, Sisters Unseen* Silver Spring, Md.: Shakti Productions. Videotape.

Ports, Suki. 1990. "Many Cultures, Many Approaches." In ACT UP, 107–12.

"Prenatal Care Affects IQ, Study of Twins Determines." 1997. *Washington Post* July 31:A11.

Purdy, Laura M. 1996. *Reproducing Persons: Issues in Feminist Bioethics.* Ithaca: Cornell University Press.

"PWA Coalition Portfolio." 1988. In Crimp, 147–68.

Quam, Michael D. 1990. "The Sick Role, Stigma, and Pollution: The Case of AIDS." In *Culture and AIDS,* ed. Douglas Feldman, 29–44. New York: Praeger.

Rawls, John. 1971. *A Theory of Justice.* Cambridge: Harvard University Press.

Raymond, Janice G. 1994. *Women as Wombs: Reproductive Technologies and the Battle over Women's Freedom.* New York: HarperCollins.

———. 1982. "Medicine as Patriarchal Religion." *Journal of Medicine and Philosophy* 7:197–216.

Reed, Wornie L. 1981. "Suffer the Children: Some Effects of Racism on the Health of Black Infants." In Conrad and Kern, 314–26.

Rich, Adrienne. 1980. "Compulsory Heterosexuality and Lesbian Existence." *Signs* 5(4):631–60.

Rich, Spencer. 1996. "Welfare Mothers Suffer More Violent Abuse." *Washington Post* August 28:A2.

Richie, Beth [E]. 1990. "AIDS: In Living Color." In White, 182–86.

Richie, Beth E., and Valli Kanuha. 1993. "Battered Women of Color in Public Health Systems: Racism, Sexism, and Violence." In Bair and Cayleff, 288–99.

Roberts, Dorothy E. 1994. "Reconstructing the Patient: Starting with Women of Color." In Wolf, 116–43.

Roberts, Helen. 1985. *The Patient Patients: Women and Their Doctors.* London: Pandora.

Rogers, Judith G. 1996. "Pregnancy and Physical Disabilities." In Krotoski, Nosek, and Turk, 101–8.

Rome, JoAnne. 1989. Untitled. *Sinister Wisdom* 39 (Winter):35–40.

Rosenwaks, Zev, Fred Benjamin, and Martin L. Stone, eds. 1987. *Gynecology: Principles and Practice.* New York: Macmillan.

Rothman, Barbara Katz. 1989. *Recreating Motherhood.* New York: W. W. Norton & Company.

———. 1982. *In Labor: Women and Power in the Birthplace.* New York: W. W. Norton & Company.

Russell, Cristine. 1995. "Percentage of Physicians Doing Abortions Declines." *Washington Post* September 23:A3.

Ruzek, Sheryl Burt. 1978. *The Women's Health Movement.* New York: Praeger.

Saliba, Claire. 1997. "Just Say No: How the Welfare Bill Could Change the Way Teenagers Learn about Sex." *Village Voice, "Class Action"* January 21:2.

Sanchez, Rene, and Richard Morin. 1993. "Straight Talk about Being Gay." *Washington Post* April 19:A1.

Sandel, Michael. 1982. *Liberalism and the Limits of Justice.* Cambridge: Cambridge University Press.

Sanford, Linda Tschirhart, and Mary Ellen Donovan. 1984. *Women and Self-Esteem.* New York: Penguin.

Sargent, Lydia, ed. 1981. *Women and Revolution.* Boston: South End Press.

Schaefer, Carol. 1991. *The Other Mother.* New York: Soho.

Schensul, Jean J., and Barbara H. Guest. 1994. "Ethics, Ethnicity, and Health Care Reform." In Dula and Goering, 24–40.

Schnall, Peter L., and Rochelle Kern. 1981. "Hypertension in American Society: An Introduction to Historical Materialist Epidemiology." In Conrad and Kern, 97–122.

Schulman, Sarah. 1990. *People in Trouble.* New York: Plume.

Schwartz, John. 1994. "Tobacco Executive Defends Testimony." *Washington Post* June 24:A1, 3.

Schwartzberg, Steven. 1996. *A Crisis of Meaning: How Gay Men Are Making Sense of AIDS.* New York: Oxford University Press.

Scully, Diana. 1980. *Men Who Control Women's Health Care.* Boston: Houghton Mifflin.

Scully, Diana, and Pauline Bart. 1981. "A Funny Thing Happened on the Way to the Orifice: Women in Gynecology Textbooks." In Conrad and Kern, 350–55.

Sears, James T. 1991. *Growing Up Gay in the South.* Binghamton, N.Y.: Harrington Park.

Segal, Judy. 1997. "Incommensurable Discourses: Personal and Institutional Talk on Death and Dying: Toward a Rhetorical Pedagogy for Medical Humanities." College Composition and Communication Conference, Phoenix, March.

Segrest, Mab. 1994. *Memoir of a Race Traitor.* Boston: South End Press.

Seiden, Anne M. 1978. "The Sense of Mastery in the Childbirth Experience." In *The Woman Patient,* vol. 1, *Sexual and Reproductive Aspects of Women's Health Care,* ed. Malkah T. Notman and Carol C. Nadelson, 87–105. New York: Plenum.

Seldin, Donald W. 1984. "The Medical Model: Biomedical Science as the Basis of Medicine." In Lee, Estes, and Ramsay, 55–62.

"Sex Education Offers Skewed View of Sex." 1997. *Washington Blade* May 9:18.

Shaw, Susan. 1997. "Beyond Safer Sex: Challenges of the HIV Epidemic for Women." National Women's Studies Association Conference, Saint Louis, June.

Shelp, Earl E., ed. 1981. *Justice and Health Care.* Dordrecht, Reidel.

Shen, Fern. 1993. "Welts Betray Dark Side of Teen Dating." *Washington Post* July 18:A1, 16.

Sherrill, Robert. 1995. "Medicine and the Madness of the Market." *The Nation* 260.2 (January 9):45–72.

Sherwin, Susan. 1992. *No Longer Patient: Feminist Ethics and Health Care.* Philadelphia: Temple University Press.

———. 1989. "Feminist and Medical Ethics: Two Different Approaches to Contextual Ethics." *Hypatia* 4.2 (Summer):57–72.

Shreve, Anita. 1989. *Women Together, Women Alone: The Legacy of the Consciousness-Raising Movement.* New York: Viking Press.

Singer, Linda. 1993. *Erotic Welfare: Sexual Theory and Politics in the Age of Epidemic.* New York: Routledge.

Smith-Rosenberg, Carroll. 1985. *Disorderly Conduct: Visions of Gender in Victorian America.* New York: Alfred A. Knopf.

Snitow, Ann, Christine Stansell, and Sharon Thompson, eds. 1983. *Powers of Desire: The Politics of Sexuality.* New York: Monthly Review Press.

Southern Poverty Law Center. 1997. "Anti-Homosexual Crime: 'The Severity of the Violence Shows the Hatred.'" *Intelligence Report* 88 (Fall):16–17.

Spelman, Elizabeth V. 1988. *Inessential Woman.* Boston: Beacon Press.

Standing, Hilary. 1980. "'Sickness' Is a Woman's Business?: Reflections on the Attribution of Illness." In Brighton Women, 124–38.

Stark, Evan, Anne Flitcraft, and William Frazier. 1983. "Medicine and Patriarchal Violence: The Social Construction of a 'Private' Event." In Fee, 177–209.

Steinem, Gloria. 1992. *Revolution from Within.* Boston: Little, Brown.

Stern, Lawrence. 1983. "Opportunity and Health Care." *Journal of Medicine and Philosophy* 8(4):339–62.

Stewart, Jean. 1989. *The Body's Memory.* New York: St. Martin's.

"Study Supports Suspicions about C-Sections, Researchers Say." 1993. *Washington Post* January 20:A9.

"Survey Reveals Abuse of AIDS Patients." 1992. *Washington Post* April 18:A22.

"Survey Reveals Doctors Uneasy about Treating Gays." 1991. *Windy City Times* December 12.

Syme, S. Leonard, and Lisa F. Berkman. 1981. "Social Class, Susceptibility, and Sickness." In Conrad and Kern, 35–44.

Szasz, Thomas. 1974. *The Myth of Mental Illness.* New York: Perennial.

"Taking Chances with AIDS." 1997. *Washington Post* August 14:A11.

Tavris, Carol. 1992. *The Mismeasure of Woman.* New York: Simon & Schuster.

Teitelbaum, Phyllis. 1989. "Feminist Theory and Standardized Testing." In Jaggar and Bordo, 324–35.

Todd, Alexandra, and Sue Fisher. 1988. *Gender and Discourse.* Norwood, N.J.: Ablex.

Tong, Rosemarie. 1997. *Feminist Approaches to Bioethics: Theoretical Reflections and Practical Applications*. Boulder: Westview.

Treichler, Paula A. 1988a. "AIDS, Gender, and Biomedical Discourse: Current Contests for Meaning." In Fee and Fox, 190–266.

———. 1988b. "AIDS, Homophobia, and Biomedical Discourse: An Epidemic of Signification." In Crimp, 31–70.

Tronto, Joan. 1989. "Women and Caring: What Can Feminists Learn about Morality from Caring?" In Jaggar and Bordo, 172–87.

Tuana, Nancy. Forthcoming. "Fleshing Rhetoric: Speaking Bodies, Refiguring Sex/Gender." In *Rethinking Sex and Gender*, ed. Tina Chanter. Cambridge: Cambridge University Press.

Vaid, Urvashi. 1995. *Virtual Equality: The Mainstreaming of Gay and Lesbian Liberation*. New York: Anchor Books.

Valverde, Mariana. 1987. *Sex, Power, and Pleasure*. Philadelphia: New Society.

Vance, Carole S., ed. 1984. *Pleasure and Danger: Exploring Female Sexuality*. New York: Routledge.

VanDerWeele, Maribeth. 1991. "Disturbing Analysis of a National Disaster." *Chicago Sun-Times* September 15.

"Views on Gay Issues." 1993. *Washington Post* April 18.

Vobejda, Barbara. 1997. "One-fifth of Women Report Being Forced to Have Sex." *Washington Post* June 6: A24.

———. 1994. "Teens Improve on Prevention of Pregnancy." *Washington Post* June 7: A1.

Voda, Ann M., Myra Dinnerstein, and Sheryl R. O'Donnell, eds. 1982. *Changing Perspectives on Menopause*. Austin: University of Texas Press.

Walker, Lenore. 1979. *The Battered Woman*. New York: Harper.

Wallsgrove, Ruth. 1980. "The Masculine Face of Science." In Brighton Women, 228–40.

Warshaw, Carole. 1994. "Domestic Violence: Challenges to Medical Practice." In Dan, 201–18.

Watney, Simon. 1989. "AIDS, Language, and the Third World." In *Taking Liberties*, ed. Erica Carter and Simon Watney, 183–92. London: Serpents Tail.

Waxman, Barbara Faye. 1996. "Commentary on Sexual and Reproductive Health." In Krotoski, 179–92.

Weeks, Jeffrey. 1977. *Coming Out*. London: Quartet.

Weise, Elizabeth Reba, ed. 1992. *Closer to Home: Bisexuality and Feminism*. Seattle: Seal.

Weisskopf, Michael. 1992. "EPA Report Addresses 'Environmental Racism.'" *Chicago Sun-Times* January 19.

Weitz, Rose. 1991. *Life with AIDS*. New Brunswick, N.J.: Rutgers University Press.

Welner, Sandra. 1996. "Contraception, Sexually Transmitted Diseases, and Menopause." In Krotoski, 81–90.

Welsh, Patrick. 1994. "Newt is Right . . . And so is Joycelyn—The Safest Sex: Kids Know What Elders Meant." *Washington Post* December 18:C1, 4.

Wendell, Susan. 1996. *The Rejected Body: Feminist Philosophical Reflections on Disability.* New York: Routledge.

———. 1989. "Towards a Feminist Theory of Disability." *Hypatia* 4(2):104–24.

Wertz, Richard, and Dorothy Wertz. 1977. *Lying-In.* New York: Free Press.

Weston, Kath. 1991. *Families We Choose: Lesbians, Gays, Kinship.* New York: Columbia University Press.

White, Evelyn C., ed. 1990. *The Black Women's Health Book: Speaking for Ourselves.* Seattle: Seal.

White, Jonathan. 1996. "Bisexuals Who Kill." Lavender Languages and Rhetoric Conference, American University, Washington, D.C., September.

Williams, Linda. 1989. *Hard Core: Power, Pleasure, and the "Frenzy of the Visible."* Berkeley: University of California Press.

Williamson, Mildred. 1994. "Women and Children Living with HIV: Impact of Racism and Poverty." In Dula and Goering, 90–98.

Wolf, Susan M., ed. 1996. *Feminism and Bioethics: Beyond Reproduction.* New York: Oxford University Press.

Wolinsky, Howard. 1991. "Effort Urged to Curb Teen AIDS." *Chicago Sun-Times* March 14.

Woods, Kristy. 1994. "Homelessness: A Risk Factor for Poor Health." In Dula and Goering, 105–20.

Worth, Dooley. 1989. "Sexual Decision-Making and AIDS: Why Condom Promotion among Vulnerable Women Is Likely to Fail." *Studies in Family Planning* 20(6):297–307.

Young, Iris Marion. 1990. *Justice and the Politics of Difference.* Princeton: Princeton University Press.

Zarembka, Arlene. 1996. "With Health Reform, Several Problems Linger." *Washington Blade* October 11:43.

Zita, Jacquelyn N. 1988. "The Premenstrual Syndrome: Dis-easing the Female Cycle." *Hypatia* 3.1 (Spring):77–100.

Zola, Irving Kenneth. 1981. "Medicine as an Institution of Social Control." In Conrad and Kern, 511–26.

Index